The Art of Scientific Publication

Do's and Don'ts for Beginners

The Art of Scientific Publication

Do's and Don'ts for Beginners

Editor-in-Chief

Nandini Chatterjee MD FRCP(Glasgow, London) FICP
Professor
Department of Medicine
Institute of Postgraduate Medical
Education and Research (IPGMER) and SSKM Hospital
Kolkata, West Bengal, India
Ex-Editor Journal of Indian Medical Association (JIMA)
Editor-in-Chief Bengal Physician Journal
(Association of Physicians of India)

Editoral Board

Jyotirmoy Pal
Mangesh Tiwaskar
Sujoy Ghosh

Foreword

Alaka Deshpande

JAYPEE

JAYPEE BROTHERS MEDICAL PUBLISHERS
The Health Sciences Publisher
New Delhi | London

Jaypee Brothers Medical Publishers (P) Ltd

Headquarters
EMCA House
23/23-B, Ansari Road, Daryaganj
New Delhi 110 002, India
Landline: +91-11-23272143, +91-11-23272703
+91-11-23282021, +91-11-23245672
E-mail: jaypee@jaypeebrothers.com

Corporate Office
Jaypee Brothers Medical Publishers (P) Ltd.
4838/24, Ansari Road, Daryaganj
New Delhi 110 002, India
Phone: +91-11-43574357
Fax: +91-11-43574314
E-mail: jaypee@jaypeebrothers.com

Overseas Office
JP Medical Ltd.
83, Victoria Street, London
SW1H 0HW (UK)
Phone: +44-20 3170 8910
Fax: +44(0)20 3008 6180
E-mail: info@jpmedpub.com

Website: www.jaypeebrothers.com
Website: www.jaypeedigital.com

Inquiries for bulk sales may be solicited at: jaypee@jaypeebrothers.com

The Art of Scientific Publication Do's and Don'ts for Beginners / Nandini Chatterjee

First Edition: 2024

ISBN: 978-93-5696-780-9

Printed at: Sterling Graphics Pvt. Ltd.

CONTRIBUTORS

Agam Vora MBBS DETRD
MD(Tuberculosis and Chest)
Senior Consultant Pulmonologist and Director
Vora Clinic and BSES Hospital
Mumbai, Maharashtra, India

Ankit Jitani DM(Clinical Hematology)
Consultant Hematologist and
Bone Marrow Transplant Physician
Marengo CIMS Hospital
Ahmedabad, Gujarat, India

Arnab Bhattacharyya MBBS DCH
MD(General Medicine) Calcutta University
FICP
Senior Consultant
PG Teacher of DNB Course
Assistant Professor
Department of Medicine
Barasat Government Medical College
Kolkata, West Bengal, India

Aryan Prasad BTech
Student (4th year)
Computer Science and
Communication Engineering
Kalinga Institute of Industrial Technology
Bhubaneswar, Odisha, India

Atanu Chandra MD(Internal Medicine)
DNB(Internal Medicine) MRCP(UK)
Assistant Professor
Department of Internal Medicine
Bankura Sammilani Medical College
Bankura, West Bengal, India

Avijit Hazra MBBS MD(Pharmacology)
Professor
Department of Pharmacology
Institute of Postgraduate Medical
Education and Research (IPGMER)
Kolkata, West Bengal, India

Bidita Khandelwal MD(Medicine)
Professor and Ex-Head
Department of Medicine
Sikkim Manipal Institute of Medical Sciences
Gangtok, Sikkim, India

Chiranjib Bagchi DGO
MD(Pharmacology) DM(Clinical Pharmacology)
Associate Professor
Department of Clinical and
Experimental Pharmacology
Calcutta School of Tropical Medicine
Kolkata, West Bengal, India

Jyotirmoy Pal MBBS MD(General Medicine) FRCP FICP FACP WHO Fellow
Professor
Department of Medicine
College of Medicine and Sagore
Dutta Hospital
Kolkata, West Bengal, India
Dean, Indian College of Physicians (ICP)
President-Elect
Association of Physicians (API)

Mangesh Tiwaskar MBBS MD FRCP FICP
Editor-in-Chief
Journal of the Association of Physicians of India
Dr E Moses Road
Mumbai, Maharashtra, India

Nandini Chatterjee MD FRCP(Glasgow, London) FICP
Professor
Department of Medicine
Institute of Postgraduate Medical Education and Research (IPGMER) and SSKM Hospital
Kolkata, West Bengal, India
Ex-Editor Journal of Indian Medical Association (JIMA)
Editor-in-Chief Bengal Physician Journal (Association of Physicians of India)

Prakas Kumar Mandal DM(Clinical Hematology)
Professor
Hematologist, Hemato-Oncologist
Bone Marrow Transplant Physician
Department of Hematology
Nil Ratan Sircar Medical College
Kolkata, West Bengal, India

Rakesh Bhadade MBBS MD FICP(Medicine)
JT Secretary Presidents Place
Professor of Medicine
TN Medical College and BYL Nair Hospital
Mumbai, Maharashtra, India

Saibal Das MBBS MD(Pharmacology) DM(Clinical Pharmacology)
Scientist D (Medical)
ICMR–Centre for Ageing and Mental Health
Kolkata, West Bengal, India

Sanjay Bandyopadhyay MD DNB DM(Gastroenterology) MNAMS FRCP
Head
Department of Gastroenterology
ILS Hospitals, Dumdum
Kolkata, West Bengal, India

Santanu K Tripathi MBBS MD DM(Clinical Pharmacology)
Consultant
Senior Clinical Pharmacologist
Academic Dean
Professor and Head
Department of Pharmacology
Netaji Subhas Medical College and Hospital
Patna, Bihar, India

Shambo Samrat Samajdar MBBS MD DM(Clinical Pharmacology) Fellowship Respiratory and Critical Care(WBUHS) Fellow Allergy-Asthma Specialist Course (AAAAI) Diploma(Allergy Asthma Immunology) PG Diploma Endocrinology and Diabetes (RCP)
Independent Clinical, Pharmacologist and Consultant Physician
Diabetes and Allergy-Asthma Therapeutics Specialty Clinic
Kolkata, West Bengal, India

Shreyashi Dasgupta MBBS MD DM(Clinical Pharmacology)
Clinical Pharmacologist
Department of Clinical and Experimental Pharmacology
Calcutta School of Tropical Medicine
Kolkata, West Bengal, India

Sujoy Ghosh DM FRCP FACE
Professor
Department of Endocrinology
Institute of Postgraduate Medical Education and Research (IPGMER)
Kolkata, West Bengal, India

FOREWORD

Art in any form is a God's gift! Its appeal lies in its beautiful presentation.

Think of any art form... painting, sculpture, music, literature, and so on.

The experience gained in developing any art form resulted into formulation of certain framework, regulations, and scientific principles for the refinement.

The same is applicable for presentation of a scientific work.

To write it systematically and prepare it for a publication, the process is both an Art and Science.

I am really very happy that Professor Nandini Chatterjee has taken the initiative and the efforts of her team have resulted into a comprehensive monograph on **"The Art of Scientific Publication—Do's and Don'ts for Beginners"**.

Most of the aspects of scientific publication have been very lucidly explained:

- Selecting an appropriate but catchy title, abstract writing, main article with its chronological sequence, bibliography
- Various types of articles, e.g., case report, research article, review article, letter to the editor, short communication, etc.
- Selection of a suitable journal
- Requirements of a particular journal
- Ethics of publication

It is fascinating to read A to Z of a scientific publication in one book.

I appeal to all our young doctors from various disciplines of medicine to start preparing their work for publication.

Unless one takes the first step, the goal cannot be reached.

I heartily congratulate Professor Nandini Chatterjee, Professor Sujoy Ghosh, and all the contributors for the comprehensive and unique monograph.

I am sure it will inspire and guide many clinicians to share their work in an appropriate journal.

I once again congratulate all the authors of this EXCELLENT monograph.

I hope to see more such work from Professor Nandini and her esteemed team.

Alaka Deshpande MD FRCP(London) MNAMS FIMSA FICP
Past Dean, Indian College of Physicians

PREFACE

What is This Book About?

The Art of Publication is a comprehensive collection by experts in the field, which will guide the readers to prepare manuscripts effectively. Manuscript preparation, its submission, revision, and final publication is a multistep process which has been standardized over the years. The beginners need to be aware of the tricks of the trade, so to say so that the chances of rejection get diminished. There are common mistakes made in articles submitted; e.g., texts that are too wordy or too long or difficult to follow. There are grammatical, spelling, or formatting errors. At times, the content may be insufficient or not up to date. It is also common to find incomplete author details, ghost writers, and plagiarism.

This book aims to help the authors to avoid these errors and also to be aware of the standard guidelines and ethics of publication. The chapters include manuscript preparation techniques of case reports, original articles, review articles, and meta-analysis. There are tips on how to choose journals before submission and how to respond to reviewer queries.

Why do We Need This Book?

Publications are essential nowadays to promote academic and career progression. Also, they are necessary for dissemination of novel information. To identify gaps in current knowledge and plan future work.

However, the process is not easy and it has its ups and downs. One has to prepare oneself for criticism and learn to handle rejection. One must train oneself to utilize the feedback of the reviewers to revise the manuscript and send it again to another appropriate journal.

This book will be a ready reckoner for accessing basic publication guidelines. There are also some self-assessment questionnaires which may be solved for better comprehension.

The National Medical Commission (NMC) has made publications mandatory for job applications and promotions and the current postgraduate medical curriculum has stressed upon publications. Hence, I sincerely hope this book will be useful to my readers in preparing a good-quality manuscript suitable for publication.

Nandini Chatterjee MD FRCP(Glasgow, London) FICP
Professor
Department of Medicine
Institute of Postgraduate Medical
Education and Research (IPGMER) and SSKM Hospital
Kolkata, West Bengal, India

CONTENTS

Section 1: Introduction

Section 2: Manuscript Preparation

Section 3: Manuscript Submission

1

SECTION

Introduction

CHAPTER 1

Why Do We Need to Publish?

Nandini Chatterjee

INTRODUCTION

Awareness about publication of scientific work is the need of the hour. Medical science is expanding its horizons day by day and there is an emergent need of new evidences to be documented for the dissemination of knowledge.

The reasons for publishing your work are two-pronged. On one hand it benefits others; on the other, it benefits you.

HOW DOES IT BENEFIT OTHERS?

New evidence generated from research or clinical observations needs to be documented for the knowledge of a wider population. Your published paper can help in the public understanding of a research question.

Published literature in peer-reviewed journals leads to wider data sharing as well as gives credit to those who share their data.

In these days of open-access journals, there is widespread dissemination of information, and they can be reused for further experimentation.

The most important aspect of scientific documentation is that information will be preserved for posterity to compare and build upon by future researchers.

HOW DOES IT BENEFIT YOU?

The act of preparing the manuscript will help you to review and interpret your own data.

It puts your research into perspective when you compare your work with that of others.

Peer review of the paper gives insight and feedback on the accuracy and quality of your research methodology and gives direction for further advances in your work.

This is also true for other types of publications such as case reports, review articles or simply pictorial Coronal mass ejections (CMEs).

A portfolio of a large number of publications gives recognition among the peers and contributes to career advancement as you are considered for academic appointments and promotions.

Publishing helps establish you as an expert in your field and may pave the way to further acquisition of research opportunities and funding.

Performance of a researcher is evaluated on the body of work he/she produces over a period of time and not on the basis of a single study in a high impact journal or the absolute number of publications.

CONCLUSION

In a nutshell, publications are part and parcel of your academic journey, requiring a lot of patience and practice to master the art of scientific writing. It is a good idea to start early, beginning with case reports or letters to the editor and then go on to more complicated documents such as original articles.

FURTHER READINGS

1. Sage Publications. Manuscript Submission Guidelines. [online] Available from http://www.uk.sagepub.com/msg/hsr.htm#ARTICLETYPES. [Last accessed January, 2024].
2. Nature Publications. Author Resources. [online] Available from http://www.nature.com/authors/author_resources/article_types.html.

CHAPTER 2

What are the Various Types of Publications?

Nandini Chatterjee

INTRODUCTION

There are different categories of publications. Different journals may not accept all types of articles; hence, it is very important to ascertain the scope of a journal by carefully going through the website of the journal and the instructions to authors. A basic idea about the different types of publications is also necessary as we plan to pen down a manuscript.

ORIGINAL RESEARCH

This type of journal manuscript is utilized to provide documentation of data from research. It is referred to by several names—Original Article, Research Article, Research, or just Article, depending on the journal. The Original Research format is suitable for different types of studies—observational, analytical, and randomized controlled trials. These are categorized as primary literature that present new research findings or shed new light on older concepts.

They include the background of study, methodology, results, interpretation of findings, and a discussion of possible implications and limitations. Original research articles are large documents with the word limit ranging from 3,000 to 6,000 or more, depending on the journal. The STROBE (Strengthening the Reporting of Observational Studies in Epidemiology) guidelines are used for observational studies and the CONSORT (Consolidated Standards of Reporting Trials) guidelines are used for randomized controlled trials.

REVIEW ARTICLES

Review Articles provide a comprehensive summary as well as an analytical overview of existing published literature in a field. They are often written by experts in a particular arena after an invitation from the editors of a journal. There is insightful evaluation, comparison, constructive criticism, and even new recommendations or suggestions for future work. A review article comprises an abstract, body, and references ranging from 50 to 100.

These are considered as secondary literature because they do not present any new or original results. Review articles can be of three types: Literature/narrative reviews, systematic reviews, and meta-analyses. Three types of review paper are often distinguished:

1. **The Literature Review** is the standard review paper, summarizing and analyzing published literature on a general topic, reflecting the state-of-the-art and pointing out knowledge gaps.
2. **The Systematic Review** is far more structured and focuses on providing an answer to one very specific research question, in reference to primary research literature, other review papers, and possibly also gray literature.
3. **The Meta-analysis** has a similar focus to the systematic review but uses statistical methods to analyze results from several similar studies on a research question, instead of presenting and relying on the data from a single study only. The similar studies are reviewed and the results are brought together using statistical methods rather than a pure description of the single result.

The word limits of review articles are variable. For narrative reviews or literature reviews, the length could range anywhere between 8,000 and 40,000 words while systematic reviews are usually less than 10,000 words long. Some journals may also publish shorter reviews, within 3,000–5,000 words.

Reviews are read more extensively than other types of literature and are frequently cited. Thus, reviews can influence the impact factor of a journal as well as the *h*-index of an author.

CLINICAL CASE STUDY/CASE REPORT

A case report is a narrative that describes, for medical, scientific or educational purposes, a medical problem experienced by one or more patients. The advantages of case reports are that they help in pattern recognition and alert the reader to new complications, adverse reactions of drugs, or new recommendations on therapy. Writing case reports trains a beginner for manuscript preparation and publication. Moreover, they can be published within a short time.

The cases presented are usually those that have educational value and contribute significantly to the existing knowledge in the field. These are considered primary literature and usually have a word count of 1,000–1,500. For accuracy of case report writing, the CARE Guidelines, with a 13-point checklist have been devised.

CASE SERIES

This is a conglomeration of more than 4 cases but less than 10. Cases with common characteristics clinically or related to pathophysiology or therapeutic strategies may be grouped together to write a case series.

SHORT COMMUNICATIONS OR LETTERS TO THE EDITOR

These are brief write-ups that may present a reanalysis of a published article or an abridged report of research or cases. Sometimes, the author expresses an opinion, queries, or constructive criticism and at times it is likely to stimulate further research in the field. This format often has strict length limits, around 500 words. So, some detailed data may not be published until the authors write a full original research manuscript.

PICTORIALS OR CLINICAL IMAGES

Authors may publish good-quality clinical photographs of interesting cases or findings. This will help the readers in spot diagnosis by pattern recognition or first impression. The accompanying text should include a short clinical presentation and discussion.

The figures or photographs should protect the privacy and identity of the patient. Legends provided should be self-explanatory. Proper consent of the subject is mandatory.

COMMENTARY

A commentary is a narrative text with an opinionated overtone. It showcases the viewpoint of the author on a particular subject. Commentaries are short articles, usually around 1,000–1,500 words long, that highlight a previously published article or book. A perspective piece is a similar essay that presents a personal point of view evaluating widely accepted notions pertaining to a field.

BOOK REVIEW

Book review provides an insightful analysis and evaluation of a recently published scholarly book. It portrays the highlights of the book and discusses the ways it would benefit the readers. Book review is also a relatively short article and allows the readers to stay updated on new literature in the field.

CONCLUSION

Journals offer multifarious options or types of articles that may be published. It is important to decide what type of article you may choose to submit depending on your experience in scientific manuscript preparation.

It is to be kept in mind that all peer-reviewed journals may not accept all paper types. Before submission, it is imperative to go through their website meticulously where guidelines for authors are given. Most often, the journal will clearly state what type of papers they accept. Thus, choose your right journal, write a paper, and embark on the voyage through the world of academia.

FURTHER READINGS

1. Nature Publications. Author Resources. [online] Available from http://www.nature.com/authors/author_resources/article_types.html
2. Academy Health. Writing Articles for Peer-review Publications: A Quick Reference Guide. [online] Available from http://www.academyhealth.org/files/HIT/writingguide.pdf [Last accessed January, 2024].
3. Zurich-Basel Plant Science Center. Guidelines for writing a review article. [online] Available from http://ueberfachliche-kompetenzen.ethz.ch/dopraedi/pdfs/Mayer/guidelines_review_article.pdf

2

SECTION

Manuscript Preparation

CHAPTER 3

Choosing a Suitable Title and the Art of Abstract Writing

Prakas Kumar Mandal, Ankit Jitani

KEY POINTS

- Check the "Instructions to Authors" of the journal you wish to submit your research.
- The first impression that ignites interest in any reader to read a paper is its title, followed by abstract.
- The title of the scientific paper serves the purpose of a movie poster, and the abstract serves as the purpose of a trailer.
- The abstract helps the reader to understand the basic content of any research work.
- Keep a watch on the word limit.
- It must be read, reviewed, and revised by all the authors.

INTRODUCTION

"What's in a name?". This famous quote by William Shakespeare does seem to be true. The beauty of a valley, the amazing depth of the ocean and as quoted by the author, the sweet smell of a rose would remain the same, whatever term we use to call them. This appears to be seemingly true, as the actual merit does not lie in a name. Same should stand true for scientific papers where the merit lies in the scientific content and not the title of the paper. However, just like movies where posters, teasers, or trailers are required to attract an audience, the title of the scientific paper serves the purpose of a movie poster, and the abstract serves as the purpose of a trailer. The first impression that ignites interest in any reader to read a paper is its title, followed by abstract. It is sad but true that many of the readers will stop at the level of the abstract. However, a few who continue and read the whole paper, do so if they are intrigued by the title and abstract. So, I say, the abstract is the trailer of the movie.

PART I: CHOOSING A SUITABLE TITLE

WHY IS THE TITLE IMPORTANT?

The Title of the article not only develops interest in the reader but is also important for the journal editor and reviewer. The editor, based on these entities, decides whether to further process the paper or not. During the review process, it creates the much required first impression. While a reader browses through the content of the journal, the title develops interest to read the abstract and the article. Additionally, the search engine optimization searches an article based on the title and keywords. So not just for interest but to get better coverage and attract more citations it is essential to have an appropriate title for the research work.[1-5]

WHAT ARE THE DIFFERENT TYPES OF TITLES?[6]

- *Descriptive or neutral or intervention-based title*: This type of title covers the study design, methodology, and the outcome. The results and conclusions are not, however, completely revealed. It gives a glimpse of the research work to its readers and has the maximum probability of appearing in search engines and hence to be cited.[7]
  Example: *The effect of posttransplant cyclophosphamide as a graft-versus-host disease (GvHD) prophylaxis in haploidentical stem cell transplant: A randomized phase 3 clinical trial.*
- *Declarative or outcome-based title*: In this type of title, the author declares the result of the article in the title itself. This is not considered the best title as it may indicate a bias toward the author. It may also create a bias in the mind of the reader whether to browse through the abstract or not.
  Example: *Posttransplant cyclophosphamide reduces the incidence of graft-versus-host disease in haploidentical stem cell transplant.*
- *Hypothesis based or interrogative title*: This type of title reveals the research question of the articles in brief. This type of title ends with a query or a question and may be interrogative.
  Example: *Does posttransplant cyclophosphamide reduce the incidence of GvHD in haploidentical stem cell transplant?*
- *Comparative titles*: When two types of interventions are being compared, these titles can be used for the article. It gives a good glimpse of the study design and method without revealing the result.
  Example: *Comparative study on the efficacy of posttransplant cyclophosphamide versus methotrexate in reducing the incidence of GvHD in haploidentical stem cell transplant.*

HOW TO APPROACH A TITLE?

Writing the title of the paper seems easy, but it takes some effort to write a perfect title. A title should be accurate and appropriate and at the same time interesting and representative of the work being discussed in the article. The same must be meticulously written, which needs both time and energy. There are five steps to create a good title for your research article. Let's discuss the approach in a nutshell with the same example as discussed earlier.

Step 1: Laydown the key questions of your scientific research paper: You must be clear on the hypothesis of your paper and what you were trying to achieve. The answer to these questions lies in your manuscript **(Table 1)**. It is still better if you have written down the abstract and answer these questions based on your abstract.

Step 2: Identify the keywords: The answers to the above questions are reasonably long. They need to be concise. From the answers to each of the above questions, select a few most important words **(Table 2)**. This is a very important step as these are the words that a search engine looks for when it shows results to its clients. Therefore, the selection must be meticulous. You may take the help from previous similar studies done on the same topic, which appear on the search results when you browse. There is usually a limit of 3–8 keywords that most of the journals allow, and this has to be well kept in mind.

Step 3: Use these keywords to frame a title: We conducted a randomized clinical trial of 200 patients between 18 and 65 years of age who received posttransplant cyclophosphamide for prevention of GvHD in haploidentical stem cell transplant for hematological malignancies; results show reduction in the incidence of GvHD.

TABLE 1: Framing key questions and most appropriate answers to those.

Question	Answer(s)
What was your hypothesis?	My research studies the impact of posttransplant cyclophosphamide in prevention of graft-versus-host disease (GvHD) in haploidentical stem cell transplant for hematological malignancies
What was the study methodology?	It was a randomized clinical trial
Who were included in the study population?	I studied 200 patients between 18 and 65 years age who underwent haploidentical stem cell transplant for hematological malignancies
What were the results?	My study showed reduction in the incidence of GvHD in patients receiving posttransplant cyclophosphamide

TABLE 2: Identifying the keywords based on the answers given to framed questions.	
Answers	**(Important) keywords**
My research studies the impact of posttransplant cyclophosphamide in prevention of graft-versus-host disease (GvHD) in haploidentical stem cell transplant for hematological malignancies	• Posttransplant cyclophosphamide • Prevention of GvHD • Haploidentical stem cell transplant • Hematological malignancies
It was a randomized clinical trial	• Randomized clinical trial
I studied 200 patients between 18 and 65 years age who underwent haploidentical stem cell transplant for hematological malignancies	• 200 patients • 18–65 years age
My study showed reduction in the incidence of GvHD in patients receiving posttransplant cyclophosphamide	• Reduction in the incidence of GvHD

The above sentence captures the essence of the paper, but it definitely is too long to be accepted as the title. The average number of words in a research title is 16.[4,6] The above sentence needs to be polished.

Step 4: *Trim the above sentence and create a working title*: In this step, all unnecessary words must be removed, the necessary words must be rephrased to create a title which will be within the permissible word limit and find more acceptance. Also, the number of patients and age of the cohort are not essential components of the title and can be safely removed. None of the important keywords should be removed. This would result in the inability of the search engines to find the article when a reader uses certain keywords to search an article.

A randomized clinical trial of posttransplant cyclophosphamide for prevention of GvHD in haploidentical stem cell transplant for hematological malignancies; results show reduction in the incidence of GvHD.

Step 5: Rephrase the above sentence: We can now rephrase the above sentence, remove a few more words, which seem unnecessary, to make a more meaningful sentence. The methodology does not seem important.

"Posttransplant cyclophosphamide reduces the incidence of graft versus host disease in haploidentical stem cell transplant for hematological malignancies."

The result of this exercise gives us a title which is relatively short and captures all essential keywords of the research. This may increase the probability of an article being found in search engines and thus enhancing the possibility of a citation.

Writing a Subtitle

In some journal papers, a subtitle may be asked for and required. The same may be added after a colon. It is wise to have a word limit for 5–6 words for the subtitle.
Example: *Posttransplant cyclophosphamide reduces GvHD*

TIPS AND TRICKS FOR WRITING A TITLE[8,9]

After this discussion on how to approach the title, let us now outline some tips and tricks which may be helpful.

- *Describe rather than ask*: Titles that describe the hypothesis well are viewed more than those posted as a question.
- *Include all the key elements*: All keywords that are pertinent to the topic should be included in the title to enable better optimization in the search engine.
- *Avoid technical and difficult to understand terms*: Articles with a simple title may be searched by people beyond your field and newcomers. Remember that researchers may use languages other than English, and simple titles may show up in other language searches as well.
- *Be concise and specific*: Articles with shorter titles have higher probability of citations.
- *Make the title more searchable*: Using all the essential keywords does the trick.
- Avoid unnecessary abbreviations and acronyms.
- *Use important keywords at the beginning*: This also helps in better article search and attracts more reads.
- *Write title at the end*: It is important to have multiple versions of the title. These versions are preferably written at the end after formulating the abstract. Take help from your peers to select the best title.
- *Do not end your title with a full stop*: Your title is not a sentence, so do not use period at the end.

PART II: THE ART OF ABSTRACT WRITING

- *"If you can't explain it simply, you don't understand it well enough."*—Albert Einstein
- *"In writing science, the abstract is poetry, the paper is prose."*[10]

WHAT IS AN ABSTRACT?

An abstract is a concise version of a longer piece of write-up that highlights the cardinal points about the content and scope of the research work. Thus, an abstract may be considered as the preview of the research.

PURPOSE OF AN ABSTRACT

An abstract helps the reader to quickly and accurately understand the basic content of any research work.

GENERAL INFORMATION ABOUT AN ABSTRACT

- The word count of an abstract varies from 100 to 350 words.
- It may accompany the publication (e.g., papers, articles, and reports) of any kind of research work
- It may sometimes be used for presentation at symposia and conferences.

WHEN AND WHERE AN ABSTRACT IS REQUIRED?

- One may start writing an abstract prior to having a paper that serves as a proposal for any project, panels, or even articles.
- Abstract can be written after someone has finished writing the paper.

WHY IS IT IMPORTANT TO WRITE AN ABSTRACT?

By writing an abstract the author(s) is/are able to answer certain key questions pertinent to the research work; for example:

- What was done (problem statement)?
- Why was it done (objective)?
- How was it done (methodology)?
- What did you find (observations/results)?
- What does it mean to others/readers (conclusion)?

DIFFERENT TYPES OF ABSTRACT?[4,6,9,11]

Depending on the discipline and research area, there are two main types of abstract:

1. *Descriptive abstract*: They are usually used for humanities and social science papers and are usually very short (50–100 words). The descriptive abstracts have some key parts: (A) Background, (B) Purpose, (C) Particular interest/focus of paper, and (D) Overview of contents (not always included).
2. *Informative abstract*: The most abstracts are written for science or psychology reports, usually in about 200 words (may vary from 150 to 350 words). These abstracts are mostly structured (divided into different parts) or may be unstructured also (as may be asked for by certain journal). Most of the structured informative abstracts have few key parts in common; each part generally consists of 1–2 sentences. The parts include: (A) Background, (B) aim or purpose of research, (C) material

www.jhas-bhs.com

ScientificScholar® Knowledge is power — Publisher of Scientific Journals

Journal of Hematology and Allied Sciences

Original Research

A glimpse into translocation (8;21) in acute myeloid leukemia: Profile and therapeutic outcomes from a tertiary care hematology center from East India

Shuvra Neel Baul[1], Avriti Baveja[2], Prakas Kumar Mandal[1], Rajib De[3], Shyamali Dutta[3], Tuphan Kanti Dolai[3]

[1]Department of Hematology, NRS Medical College and Hospital, Kolkata, West Bengal, [2]Department of Medicine (Hematology), HIMS (Cancer Research Institute), SRHU, Dehradun, Uttarakhand, [3]Department of Haematology, NRS Medical College and Hospital, Kolkata, West Bengal, India.

***Corresponding author:**
Avriti Baveja,
Department of Medicine (Hematology), HIMS (Cancer Research Institute), SRHU, Dehradun, Uttarakhand, India.
avritibaveja@gmail.com

Received : 06 January 2022
Accepted : 08 June 2022
Published : 29 October 2022

DOI
10.25259/JHAS_1_2022

Quick Response Code:

ABSTRACT

Objectives: Translocation (8;21) is a RUNX1-RUNX1T1 fusion transcript, a favorable risk cytogenetic abnormality with a variable clinicopathological profile. However, there is a paucity of data on the outcomes of acute myeloid leukemia (AML) with t(8;21) from East India. This report is an analysis of data of AML with t(8;21) at our center.

Material and Methods: *De novo* AML patients with the presence of t(8;21) cytogenetic abnormality from 2015 to 2019 were analyzed for clinical, pathological, and molecular characteristics and were compared with treatment outcomes. Relapse-free survival (RFS) and overall survival (OS) were determined using Kaplan–Meier curves.

Results: Twenty-nine patients (10%) with *de novo* AML had t(8;21) with 18 male patients and a median age of 20 years. Aberrant expression of CD19, CD56, and CD7 expressions was noted in 44.8%, 17.24%, and 10.29% of patients, respectively. Additional cytogenetic abnormality was observed in 31.03%. CD19 had an 80% correlation with the occurrence of C-kit status. High-dose induction therapy had complete remission rates of 100%. The median duration of follow-up was 287.5 days. The presence of myeloid sarcoma (MS) and C-kit positivity had inferior OS and RFS ($P < 0.05$). The dose of cytosine arabinoside, given in consolidation of 3 g/m^2 and 1.5 g/m^2, had a median OS of 758 and 479 days ($P = 0.661$) and median RFS of 348 and 150 days ($P = 0.002$), respectively. In the group that received intensive therapy, by the end of 3 years, only 15.7% of patients remain in remission.

Conclusion: AML with t(8;21) is seen in young patients with a positive correlation between CD 19 with C-kit positivity. The presence of MS and C-kit positivity endowed inferior OS and RFS. Cytosine arabinoside consolidation in a dose of 3 g/m^2 offered an advantage in median RFS.

Keywords: Acute myeloid leukemia, Cytosine arabinoside, t(8;21)

FIG. 1: Example of a structured informative abstract from an original article.
Source: Reproduced with permission from Baul SN et al.(2022)[12]

and method (methodology), (D) findings/results, (E) conclusion, and (F) recommendations (or "implications", may not be relevant; thus not necessary in all cases). In some journals, both "A" and "B" are combined together and written as "Objective(s)" as shown in **Figure 1**.

PARTS OF THE ABSTRACT (FIG. 1)

Purpose or statement of problem: Try to state the primary objectives, aims, and scope of the study or, as in review papers, briefly state the reason as to why you have written the manuscript.

Materials and Methods (approach/methodology): Clearly mention the techniques used in your research. In case of nonexperimental works (e.g., review papers), briefly describe the sources and how you used them.

Results (findings): Briefly describe the results (original research/case series) or the interpretation of sources (review articles). Mention the limitations of your research study.

CONCLUSION

How do you relate your study results to the purpose of your investigations? Also mention its future implication, if any. And, sometimes may be associated with some suggestions and/or recommendations based on your results and conclusion.

DIFFERENT STRATEGIES OF WRITING ABSTRACT FROM THE MAIN TEXT[2,4,6,9,11]

- *Option A (cut and paste approach)*: Read your draft and highlight very carefully the salient points. Cut and paste these highlighted areas, rearrange by adding or removing alphabets/word(s), and organize as per the criteria of any journal you have in your mind.
- *Option B (write afresh a complete and concise account of the whole research/work)*: Highlight the key areas to be kept and remove/delete the unimportant parts selectively. Edit and revise it repeatedly, then divide it into parts (structures) to the specifications of the call.
- *Option C (component outline approach)*: *Very useful in writing structured abstracts. From the very beginning, start writing the different parts of the* abstract. Revise and edit to make it a cohesive account of the whole work. Select words to make the abstract flow and flawless.

FORMATION OF AN UNSTRUCTURED ABSTRACT (FIG. 2)

In all sense, the same or similar steps are followed as in case of writing a structured abstract; the only/major difference is, it is not divided into parts. The easiest way to write is, first follow the structured approach, then delete/

Title: Hematuria in a young severe hemophilia patient – A case report on a rare radiological finding

ABSTRACT

Renal ectopia or ectopic kidney is one of the common renal anomalies in which there is faulty migration of the fetal pelvis during the embryonic period. Hemophilia is an inherited coagulation disorder characterized by recurrent and spontaneous bleeding due to a deficiency of clotting factor VIII or IX. Clotting factor concentrates are used as standard therapy for the management of bleeding episodes. Hematuria is the presence of blood in urine that is either visible to the naked eye (macroscopic) or nonvisible (microscopic). Common etiologies of hematuria include congenital anomalies, calculus, inflammation, and infectious and malignancy of the renal and urogenital tract. Here, we present a 14-year-old male with severe hemophilia A who presented with severe pain abdomen and hematuria. On evaluation, he was found to have a left-sided ectopic kidney. In addition to the overdue discovery of the left-sided ectopic kidney, there is the coexistence of a bleeding disorder which may pose a challenge in the patient's management.

Keywords: Severe hemophilia; Hematuria; Renal ectopia

FIG. 2: Example of an unstructured informative abstract from a case report.[13]

Source: Reproduced with permission from Roy S et al.(2023)[13]

remove the subheadings and assemble the sentences accordingly. However, it must essentially have all same theme as a structured abstract and bear the same meaning. These types of abstracts are mostly required for the case reports and review articles of few journals.

HOW DOES AN ABSTRACT DIFFER FROM AN INTRODUCTION?[6,11]

Authors, especially the beginners, are many a time get confused about the difference between an abstract and an introduction. **Table 3** briefly describes the salient features that differentiate these two in a research paper.

4-C'S OF ABSTRACT WRITING[2,6,11]

1. *Complete*—the abstract must cover all major parts of the research/study
2. *Concise*—it must be very precise; avoid unnecessary information
3. *Clear*—clearly readable; avoid jargons
4. *Cohesive*—should flow smoothly and precisely flawless

One should always try to satisfy all 4-C's to get one of the best write-ups.

3-'R' RULE (REREAD, REVIEW, AND REVISE)[2,6,11]

1. *Read*—the main points of the manuscript repeatedly and write it in such a way that it is clearly understandable even to an educated nonexpert.
2. *Review*—the abstract for accuracy, especially the result section about the data and statistics.
3. *Revise*—it to make it flawless.

TABLE 3: Differences between abstract and introduction of the main text in the manuscript.

Abstract	Introduction
An abstract is the essence of the whole paper/ manuscript	As the name indicates, it introduces the scientific paper/manuscript
It covers the following academic elements: • Background • Aim or purpose of research • Material and method (methodology) • Findings/results • Conclusion • Recommendations (or "implications"; may not be relevant, thus not necessary in all cases)	It covers the following elements: • Background • Purpose • Proposition (also called "point of view") • Outline of key issues • Scope ("not" always relevant)
Summarizes briefly the whole manuscript/paper including the conclusions	Introduces the paper and open up the key issues for discussion

DO'S AND DON'TS OF WRITING AN ABSTRACT

- Check the "Instructions to Authors" of the journal you wish to submit your research.
- Use complete sentences
- Use active voice (rather than passive voice)
- Try to avoid contractions (couldn't, didn't, etc.)
- Try to avoid personal opinions.

CHECKLIST BEFORE SUBMISSION

- Make sure it is within the word limit.
- Language is understandable by a nonspecialist
- It is read, reviewed, and revised by all the authors.

REFERENCES

1. Nair LB, Gibbert M. What makes a good title and how does it matter for citations? A review and general model of article title attributes in management science. Scientometrics. 2016;107(3):1331-59.
2. Dewan P, Gupta P. Writing the title, abstract and introduction: Looks matter! Indian Pediatr. 2016;53:235-41.
3. Bavdekar SB. Formulating the right title for a research article. J Assoc Physicians India. 2016;64:53-6.
4. Badri T. Writing the title, abstract, and keywords for a medical article: to be concise and accurate. Tunis Med. 2019;97(7):865-9.
5. Grant MJ. What makes a good title? Health Info Libr J. 2013;30(4):259-60.
6. Tullu MS. Writing the title and abstract for a research paper: Being concise, precise, and meticulous is the key. Saudi J Anaesth. 2019;13:S12-S17.
7. Njire Braticevic M, Babic I, Abramovic I, Jokic A, Horvat M. Title does matter: a cross-sectional study of 30 journals in the Medical Laboratory Technology category. Biochem Med (Zagreb). 2020;30(1):010708.
8. Annesley TM. The title says it all. Clin Chem. 2010;56:357-60.
9. Bahadoran Z, Mirmiran P, Kashfi K, Ghasemi A. The Principles of Biomedical Scientific Writing: Title. Int J Endocrinol Metab. 2019;17(4):e98326.
10. Weissmann G. Writing science: the abstract is poetry, the paper is prose. FASEB J. 2008;22:2601-4.
11. Writing an abstract. Writing center learning guide. Copyright: The University of Adelaide 2014. [online] Available from http://writingcenter.unlv.edu/writing/abstract.html [Last accessed January, 2024].
12. Baul SN, Baveja A, Mandal PK, De R, Dutta S, Dolai TK. A glimpse into translocation (8;21) in acute myeloid leukemia: Profile and therapeutic outcomes from a tertiary care hematology center from East India. J Hematol Allied Sci. 2022;2:85-90.
13. Roy S, Ghosh K, Mandal PK. Hematuria in a young severe hemophilia patient – A case report on a rare radiological finding. J Hematol Allied Sci. 2023. [Article in press].

CHAPTER 4

How to Write a Case Report?

Nandini Chatterjee

INTRODUCTION

The advent of Evidence-based Medicine spelled the doom of narrative scientific publication, which is epitomized by case reports. However, it must be remembered that knowledge about the dangerous effects of thalidomide, or the occurrence of human immunodeficiency virus (HIV) infection coincident with various infections or cancers was first documented by the humble case report.

HOW OLD IS THE CASE REPORT?

The earliest case reports date back to 1600 BC, named the Edwin Smith Papyrus recovered from Egypt. There are 48 cases discussing injuries or disorders of the head and upper torso.

Next recovered were the Hippocratic case histories in 400 BC, characterized by objective description of findings and observation of the course of the disease processes. Subsequent texts over time were clinical descriptions with personalized, dramatic presentations, as in the Galenic Case reports. From the 19th century, texts became more technical, with the categorization of the content into well-coordinated sections.[1-3]

SO, WHAT IS A CASE REPORT?

A case report is a narrative that describes, for scientific or educational purposes, clinical presentations and management of individual patients.[4]

WHY SHOULD IT BE WRITTEN?[5,6]

The main function of a case report is to help in pattern recognition.

It is an excellent tool for problem-based learning, which will help the reader to recognize similar signs and symptoms when one faces a similar case in one's daily practice.

It can also sensitize the reader to novel therapies, adverse effects of drugs, or newer complications of some diseases.

New hypotheses may be contemplated and could then be tested with advanced research methods.

Another advantage of the case report is the cost, as often the necessary work is performed in the clinical setting without specific funding.

The time span from observation to publication is also shorter than for other kinds of studies.

This is encouraging for the beginners who have embarked tentatively on the path of scientific documentation.

Writing case reports is a great way to practice manuscript preparation and gives initial exposure to the steps of publication.

WHAT ARE THE PITFALLS OF A CASE REPORT?[7]

The observer's personal experience leads to subjectivity that might bias the interpretation of the observation (i.e., information bias). Moreover, there is no possibility to establish cause–effect relationship from an uncontrolled observation.

The retrospective design may increase the chances of missing out relevant data. Recall bias, a common occurrence, might prevent one from getting the necessary information from the patient or relatives.

Thus, the evidence level is low, and it has poor citation value.

WHAT ARE THE TYPES OF CASE REPORTS?

A case report may describe:

- An unusual manifestation of a well-known disease
- A diagnostic or ethical dilemma
- An outcome of a novel treatment
- A peculiar complication of a disease
- Adverse or beneficial effects of drugs

What is important, is the educational value of the case.

WHAT ARE THE COMPONENTS OF A CASE REPORT?[8]

While writing a case report, it is important to divide the text into sections or components. Care must be taken to adhere to the word limit, for most of the journals it is 1,000–1,500 words. This excludes the abstract and references. One must read instructions to authors about the Font, Spacing, Table or Figure number, and the referencing/Citation methods.

The components of the case report may vary from journal to journal. However, the general components are:

- Title
- Abstract
- Introduction
- Case report
- Discussion
- Conclusion

However, the first task is to decide the title.

Title

The title should be concise, informative, and relevant to the subject.

The ideal title should attract the reader's attention and state the focus on a particular issue, without being too dramatic. It should mention the primary diagnosis or the intervention applied.

Abstract

An abstract is a brief summary which may be structured/unstructured. The structured abstract is given more in original articles and is usually limited to 50–100 words. It briefly describes the clinical presentation, final diagnosis, and the learning points of the case. Abstract is followed by 3–4 keywords, widely accepted terms are to be used. They help in locating information from a search engine, some journals specify to use MeSH (Medical Subject Headings) words.

Introduction

The introduction touches upon the background of the case with a brief literature review.

It is important to highlight why the case is unique or how it is relevant to daily clinical practice.

Case Report

Thereafter, we come to the Case description. This includes the history, examination, followed by the differential diagnosis.

Exclusion of differentials through clinical analysis, along with diagnostic tools utilized, should be mentioned.

Description of laboratory test results, imaging, or questionnaires as well as diagnostic challenges faced while dealing with the case (e.g., financial, language/cultural) adds to the unfolding of the final diagnosis.

This section can include tables of both measured values with normal ranges of tests.

Figures/photos may be added with detailed legends later.

A timeline, providing the chronological order of events up to the present, is also a helpful accompaniment to the descriptive text.

Next, we describe the treatment strategy, whether it was drug therapy, surgical or preventive care. Dosage, strength, and duration of pharmacotherapy along with any adverse events need to be quoted.

The author should ensure that all the relevant details are included and unnecessary ones excluded.

Lastly, the clinical course of follow-up visits is to be described. One has to include clinician and patient-assessed outcomes, follow-up investigations, and therapeutic compliance. Any adverse events can also be mentioned.

Discussion

The discussion will summarize the case and clarify the key issues.

It is important to justify the uniqueness of the case. Further elaboration includes comparison with other published literature and some light may be shed on the strengths and limitation of management.

CONCLUSION

In conclusion, the learning points of the case are to be highlighted. Any recommendation, future research, or basic science investigation that could hasten diagnosis and management may be suggested.

The CARE guidelines have been formulated to provide tools to inform and simplify the process of writing accurate and transparent case reports. It strives to improve health research reporting. There is a 13-point checklist that may be downloaded from the internet for enhancing the accuracy of manuscript writing.

PRACTICAL TIPS

It is always a good idea to discuss with other authors. A manuscript needs to be modified many times before it is ready for publication.

One has to avoid long phrases and repetition and simple words are to be used. Also grammar, syntax, and spellings are to be checked. There are specific software available for this.

It is vital to respect word length and avoid plagiarism. Most journals want the plagiarism to be less than 10–15%. Nowadays all submitted papers are screened with updated plagiarism check software.

WHAT ABOUT THE PHOTOGRAPHS OF SUBJECTS?

- Face of subject or eyes are to be covered.
- Written consent is mandatory.

- If the photograph has already been published elsewhere—acknowledgment and permission from copyright holder is to be taken.
- Creative Commons Attribution (CCA) license is a license where photos or figures are in the public domain and may be shared or utilized without permission. One has to check whether a particular site has the CCA license if any material is to be shared.[9]

WHAT ARE LEGENDS?

Legends are brief texts explaining the figures/findings in a photograph/investigations.

Detailed description for histopathology slide photographs is required.

ACKNOWLEDGMENT

At the end of the write-up an Acknowledgment may be added.

Administrative support, technical assistance, proofreading, and fund acquisition which are not considered criteria for authorship may be acknowledged at the end of the article.

REFERENCES

Reference section is a vital part of the manuscript that is often neglected. The references listed at the end of the case report should be relevant and provide additional updates for readers interested in more detailed information.

References should be around 10–15 usually, but this number may vary according to the journal concerned and is categorically mentioned in the instructions to the author.

One has to follow citation guidelines for the journal. Usually, the Vancouver style or Harvard style is used.

WHAT IS A CASE SERIES?

Though there is a lack of a clear definition and it varies from journal to journal, the standard accepted one is—a case series comprises more than 4 cases, less than 10. These are a conglomeration of cases with common characteristics clinically or related to pathophysiology or therapy.

However as these are uncontrolled and do not have a study design or research question, they are not considered as original studies. Their evidence value is also considered subjective.

HOW TO CHOOSE THE JOURNAL?

Case reports may or may not be published by certain journals. One has to get prior information about the scope of the journal before submission. Examples of journals that accept case reports are:

- BMJ Case Reports
- European Journal of Case Reports
- Journal of Medical Case Reports
- Journal of Post Graduate Medicine
- JIMA/JAPI/Bengal Physician Journal

Before submission also find out about indexing status, impact factor, and submission or processing fees.

WHAT TO DO DURING SUBMISSION?

The following documents are to be submitted along with the main manuscript.

- *Covering letter*—addressed to the editor of the journal
- *Title page*—contains the title of the case with the names, affiliations, and contact details of the authors. The order of authorship needs to be decided by discussion amongst all authors. The corresponding author should be separately mentioned, as he/she will be responsible for replying to all the queries during peer review and also for supplying all relevant documents.
- *Copyright form*—downloaded from the journal website. It transfers the copyright of the article to the journal. It is to be signed by all authors with date mentioned.
- *Informed consent form*—duly signed by patient or the guardian
- *Ethics committee approval letter*—if required by the journal. Often it is not required for case reports.

Once the case is put for peer review, the referee may send queries or a critical appraisal of the article. The corresponding author needs to respond to each query and highlight the changes that are made in the body text according to the reviewers' comments.

To conclude, writing case reports is a good way to practice the art of manuscript preparation for beginners. It trains us to follow the steps of scientific reporting and adds to the experience of submission of an article and responding to queries. It is also a time-tested means of problem-based learning, which helps in daily practice and standard patient care.

REFERENCES

1. Nissen T, Wynn R. The recent history of the clinical case report: a narrative review. J R Soc Med Short Rep. 2012;3:87-7.
2. Allen JP. The art of medicine in ancient Egypt. The Metropolitan Museum of Art, New York, New Haven and London: Yale University Press; 2005.

3. Álvarez Millán C. Graeco-Roman case histories and their influence on Medieval Islamic clinical accounts. Soc Hist Med. 1999;12(1):19-43.
4. Chelvarajah R, Bycroft J. Writing and publishing case reports: The road to success. Acta Neurochir (Wien). 2004;146:313-6.
5. Warner JO. Case reports-what is their value? Pediatr Allergy Immunol. 2005;16:93-4.
6. Petrusa ER, Weiss GB. Writing case reports: An educationally valuable experience for house officers. J Med Educ. 1982;57:415-76.
7. Mason RA. The case report – an endangered species? [Editorial]. Anesthesia. 2001;56: 99-102.
8. Hurwitz B. Form and representation in clinical case reports. Lit Med. 2006;24:216-40.
9. UNESO. The Creative Commons licenses. [online] Available from https://en.unesco.org/open-access/creative-commons-licenses [Last accessed January, 2024].

CHAPTER 5

How to Write an Original Article?

Sujoy Ghosh

INTRODUCTION

In the dynamic realm of medical research, the ability to pen an original and impactful research article holds immense significance. Such articles not only contribute to the collective knowledge of the medical community but also shape the course of scientific progress. This comprehensive guide delves into the essential components required to create an original research article that stands out.

From formulating a compelling research question to designing methodologies and presenting findings with precision, this guide offers a comprehensive approach to creating an understanding of the art of writing an original research article.

Moreover, we will delve into the significance of clear and concise writing, along with the proper use of references, ensuring that your article not only presents insights but also contributes to the broader medical audience. This article also gives general tips in sections and checklists for authors to verify each section of its excellence.

PRIMARY COMPONENT OF A RESEARCH ARTICLE

A good research paper focuses on a single research subject. The basic organizing principle of the study is the research question. What is a solid research question? The most important characteristics are: (i) specificity, (ii) uniqueness or originality, and (iii) general applicability to a large scientific audience. The research question should be specific rather than just defining a broad field of study. A study need not be an entirely new territory; rather, it should add to the existing knowledge in a beneficial way.[1]

STRUCTURE OF A RESEARCH ARTICLE (BOX 1)

After defining the research question, an original research paper can be written in a certain, preferred manner. The format usually adopted is called IMRAD [Introduction, Methods, Results, (and) Discussion] structure. Introduction, methods, results, and discussion are together referred to by the abbreviation IMRAD. The IMRAD framework aids in the elimination of unwanted details and enables the clear and orderly presentation of relevant data.[2,3] The "uniform requirements for manuscripts submitted to biomedical journals"[4] also recommend the IMRAD format.

Introduction

The introduction's goal is to capture the reader's attention by providing enough information to outline the problem or topic of the piece. The introduction should be brief, straightforward, and to the point. The introduction

BOX 1 Key messages for structuring an original article.

Introduction:
- Explain the problem's significance
- Identify gaps in current knowledge
- State the study's objective

Methods:
- Describe the study's process
- Explain the plan followed
- Discuss the group under study
- Clarify the method of selecting participants
- If any special methods were used, mention them
- Detail the focus of the study
- Explain how information was collected
- Describe the process of result analysis

Results:
- Present data collection and participant recruitment details
- Describe the characteristics of participants
- Outline key findings related to the main research question
- Share any additional findings

Discussion:
- Summarize crucial findings
- Compare results with previous research
- Discuss potential impacts on policies and practices
- Analyze the study's strengths and limitations
- Propose potential areas for future research

has four parts: (i) A quick review of the main topic, (ii) problems in past studies, (iii) the study's goal, and (iv) its scope.[5]

Start with a concise topic overview, supported by key references. Highlight issues in previous research to emphasize the study's importance. Clarify the study's purpose and how it adds to knowledge. End with a brief paragraph outlining what the study covers and how it is organized. Introduction should end with the objective of the study.

Objective

The objective of the study must include the population studied, intervention used, comparison group if any, outcome measured, and timeline of the study, which can be abbreviated as PICOT. The other commonly used term for objective is SMART (specific, measurable, achievable, relevant, and timebound).

Checklist for Introduction

- Are the objectives well defined?
- Has the significance of the study been appropriately highlighted?
- Does the study address a novel subject matter?
- Have prior works on the topic been cited sufficiently?

Methodology

It is essential to provide readers with ample details about how the study was conducted, allowing them to replicate it, if desired. This requires being specific, using technical language, and offering a level of detail that captures the study's intricacies. Describe the environment where the study took place, define the study population, outline the approach used to select samples, elaborate on the tools and instruments employed, explain how data was gathered, and detail the strategies employed for analyzing the collected information. It is important to consider that all the methods mentioned in this section should be entirely relevant to satisfying the objectives of the study; do not detail any irrelevant methods that might have been part of the study. This comprehensive approach ensures that the study's procedures are transparent and reproducible. Provide a detailed study design description, covering control specifics (if relevant) and randomization type/method, and a brief explanation of the statistical approaches adopted for data analysis in separate paragraphs.

Ethical Consideration

This section should encompass informed consent, ethical committee approval, funding source, conflict of interest disclosure, and compliance with the Declaration of Helsinki for animal studies.

Checklist for Methodology

- Have the study population details been provided sufficiently?
- Is the description of methods clear enough for experiment reproduction?
- Is the study design easily comprehensible?
- Have the statistical methods been adequately covered?
- Have ethical considerations been properly addressed?

Results

The results section is generally direct and factual. It must present all results pertinent to the research question, offering detailed figures such as counts and percentages.

Results contain two fundamental parts, the presentation of data and analysis of the results.

The outcomes from all employed methods should be organized and delivered systematically. You can display these results through text, tables, or graphs but refrain from duplicating data. Arrange the data logically, which might differ from the order of your work. Ensure that your results are expressed with clarity, precision, and no ambiguity. If there are definite numerical figures to support proportions, avoid vague terms like "most", "some", "probably", etc. Only include pertinent results aligned with the study's goal, avoiding irrelevant outcomes that could divert the reader's focus.

Analysis of Results

Examining the results entails employing statistical analysis to derive an objective validation or rejection of the hypothesis posited in the introduction. In studies involving comparisons, each individual comparison must be accompanied by its distinct statistical evaluation. In scientific pursuits, precision is the key. However, in biological sciences, measurements are inherently imprecise. Employing statistics judiciously emerges as the optimal means to encapsulate and convey this inherent variability accurately.

Checklist for Results

- Can readers understand the results from the given data?
- Is the information clear and not puzzling?
- Are there enough controls in place?
- Do the statistical methods fit the study well?

Discussion

Begin the discussion with a summary of key findings from the results section. Thoroughly discuss and compare each obtained result with relevant previous studies, logically and clearly. Explain any differences from earlier findings.

Avoid repeating points and opinions. Address each issue once. Remain neutral in opinions. Highlight all important past studies, regardless of their outcomes.

Study's Strengths and Weaknesses

Dedicate a paragraph to outlining the strengths and novel findings of the study. Follow with another paragraph detailing limitations, drawbacks, and potential ways to mitigate these in future research.

Recommendations

Offer recommendations based on study outcomes.

Checklist for Discussion

- Are all the results adequately commented upon?
- Has the rationale for the study's differences from existing literature been explained?
- Are potential issues and limitations of the study discussed?
- Do the conclusions align well with the results?

Summary

Summary can exist as an individual section or the concluding paragraph within the Discussion. Emphasize the most crucial discoveries of the study. This section acts as the key takeaway and condenses the entirety of the research. It goes beyond the abstract, functioning as an expanded conclusion that rationalizes and clarifies the study's ultimate deduction.

Abstract

Abstracts come in two forms: Free form or structured with subheadings. Always stick to the format guided by the publisher. A regular abstract includes introduction (background, question, or hypothesis), methods, results, conclusions, and implications. Initiate your abstract by presenting the study's background and the question posed and then outline your study methods. Subsequently, emphasize the main results, while minimizing the inclusion of raw data. Conclude by addressing the posed questions and summarizing the core message.

Title

The title must be informative, precise, encompassing, and accurate, effectively outlining the article's content. It should encapsulate substantial information using minimal words. Ideally, it should indicate the primary research topic and, if possible, the study type. The title ought to indicate the subject matter, steering clear of conclusions. Regular reconsideration and assessment of the title are recommended, and upon paper completion, the final title becomes the concluding sentence.

References

Styles: Two commonly used referencing styles are the alphabetical (Harvard) and the Vancouver system, with the latter being more prevalent in medical journals.[6] In the Vancouver system, references are arranged numerically based on their order of appearance in the text and are indicated in the text using numbers.

Each journal employs its specific reference style, as outlined in the "Instructions to Authors". It is advisable to carefully follow these instructions and review a recent issue of the journal to match its referencing style. Maintain consistency in the presentation and arrangement of all references. Favor recent references over older ones.

References must be used thoughtfully. Essential claims, methodologies, and employed tools should be referenced. Yet, unless the paper serves as a comprehensive review, there is no necessity for an exhaustive compilation of references.

Tables

Tables serve two main objectives: (i) Presenting content without necessitating text reading, and (ii) offering easily digestible results. An effective table should act as a standalone communication unit, both informative and intelligible. It should convey maximal information using minimal words, supplying additional insights not found in the text to avoid redundancy.

Creating a Well-designed Table

A well-constructed table requires arranging data in a meaningful sequence, excluding insignificant values and trimming superfluous language. Keep headings concise to prevent repetition and ensure simplicity, clarity, and easy comprehension. Tables should be compact, preventing the fragmentation of related data, so that all pertinent information can be found within a single table.

General Tips

Tables comparing groups must incorporate specific statistical analysis. Abbreviations, if utilized, should be clarified in a footnote, unless previously defined in the text or an abbreviation list. Tables usually follow references, each on a separate page, labeled with a number and title. It is imperative to confirm the correct table number placement in the text. When deciding between presenting data as a table or as a graph, prioritize the reader's need—opt for a graph for general trends and a table for precise values.

Illustrations and Figures

The aim of an illustration or figure is to facilitate easy understanding and enhance retention. The purpose is to convey clear information. Designing such visuals calls for simplicity, steering clear of intricate details and unnecessary elements. Renowned graphics software, although widely used, often cater to nonscientific graphics, leading to visuals more suitable for business presentations. Avoiding features like three-dimensional bars or pie charts is recommended. To ensure the quality of presentation in a peer-reviewed journal, refer to applicable advice.[7] It is important to avoid repetition and contradictions with textual or tabular content. Opting for colors suitable for photocopying, such as avoiding pale shades, can enhance reproduction quality.

General Tips

Confirm that figure numbers match their location in the text. Avoid placing the legend above or below the figure as a graphic. Legends should complement the text, avoiding redundancy. Prevent undue distraction from the text by keeping legends concise.

CRAFTING EFFECTIVE WRITING

Constructing Sentence Structure

Each sentence should encapsulate a solitary idea. Nurturing writing proficiency involves studying well-crafted papers. The keystones to accomplished writing are simplicity and lucidity.[8]

To sidestep writing pitfalls, avoid:

- Ambiguity
- Repetition
- Wordiness (unnecessary word use)
- Exaggerated writing (asserting excessive significance)
- Using special terminologies (words meant for specific groups)

Constructing Paragraph Structure

Commonly, a paragraph begins with a topic sentence that introduces its essence. Subsequently, information, data, or ideas follow, concluding with an apt ending sentence, if warranted.

COMMON ERRORS OBSERVED IN MANUSCRIPTS

- Failing to define the research question
- Presenting an unclear or vague paper objective
- Exhibiting a disorganized paper structure
- Disregarding the journal's author instructions

- Exceeding the stipulated word limit
- Elaborating extensively on the literature in the Introduction
- Insufficiently detailing methods, interventions, and instruments
- Duplicating results in both tables and text
- Including elaborate tables for results unrelated to the primary research question
- Insufficiently supporting key arguments with appropriate references in the Introduction and Discussion.
- Citing outdated or inaccessible references
- Failing to address the research question in the Discussion
- Exaggerating the implications of results without acknowledging study limitations in the discussion
- Demonstrating subpar English language proficiency in the paper

REFERENCES

1. Perneger TV, Hudelson PM. Writing a research article: Advice to beginners. Int J Qual Health Care. 2004;16(3):191-2.
2. Sollaci LB, Pereira MG. The introduction, methods, results, and discussion (IMRAD) structure: A fifty-year survey. J Med Lib Assoc. 2004;92(3):364-71. [Erratum in: J Med Lib Assoc. 2004;92(4):506.]
3. Day RA. The origins of the scientific paper: The IMRAD format. Am Med Writers Assoc J. 1989;4(2):16-8.
4. Uniform requirements for manuscripts submitted to biomedical journals: Writing and editing for biomedical publication. J Pharmacol Pharmacother. 2010;1(1):42-58.
5. Shokeir AA. How to write a medical original article: Advice from an editor. Arab J Urol. 2014;12(1):71-8.
6. Grange RI, Vale J, Williams G, Whitfield HN. Medical writing. BJU Int. 2004;94(2):225-31.
7. Grange RI. Saving time, effort and tears: A guide to presenting results. Br J Urol. 1998 Feb;81(2):335-9.
8. Grange R. The use (and misuse) of English in urological papers. Arab J Urol. 2011;9(1):63-5.

CHAPTER 6

How to Write a Review Article?

Shambo Samrat Samajdar, Sanjay Bandyopadhyay

INTRODUCTION

In the ever-evolving landscape of health sciences, the role of review articles has become increasingly pivotal. Clinicians and medical researchers alike frequently turn to these comprehensive syntheses for updating their knowledge and guiding their clinical practice.[1] Review articles serve not only as a cornerstone for developing guidelines but also as a vital resource for institutions providing financial support for further research. Their growing importance underscores the need for high-quality, well-constructed reviews that effectively communicate valuable findings and insights. Historically, the quality of review articles has been a subject of scrutiny. Studies, such as Murlow's evaluation of review articles published in the mid-1980s, have highlighted a common shortfall in adhering to rigorous scientific standards.[2] This concern led to the development of guidelines like the QUOROM (QUality of Reporting of Meta-analyses) statement and its successor,[3] PRISMA (Preferred Reporting Items for Systematic Reviews and Meta-Analyses),[4] which set benchmarks for reporting meta-analyses of randomized controlled studies.

Review articles are broadly categorized into narrative and systematic reviews. Narrative reviews offer a broad-spectrum view in an easily digestible format, allowing for a comprehensive consideration of the subject matter. Systematic reviews, on the other hand, are the gold standard in review articles. They are characterized by detailed, comprehensive literature surveys with minimal author bias and can be further subdivided into qualitative and quantitative reviews, with the latter often involving meta-analysis.[5]

The impetus behind writing a review article is fundamentally to create a coherent synthesis of the best literature sources on a significant research inquiry or topic. This process involves identifying key questions, employing meticulous methods to find and select high-quality research, and synthesizing the varied research findings. The time spent in the initial phases of determining the focus and consulting with peers is an investment in ensuring the review's relevance and depth.[6]

Adhering to the PRISMA statement's 27-item checklist can guide authors in crafting review articles that are not only scientifically robust but also clear and comprehensive.[6] **Table 1** outlines the PRISMA statement, a 27-item checklist designed to improve the reporting of systematic reviews and meta-analyses.

TABLE 1: Concise format to identify the article as a systematic review.

Item	Description
Title	Identify the article as a systematic review, meta-analysis, or both
Summary	Write a structured summary including background, objectives, data sources, study eligibility criteria, participants, treatments, study appraisal and synthesis methods, results, limitations, conclusions, implications, and registration number
Introduction	*Rationale:* Explain the rationale for the review in the context of existing knowledge
	Objectives: Provide an explicit statement of questions with reference to participants, interventions, comparisons, outcomes, and study design (PICOS)
Methods	*Protocol and registration:* Indicate if a review protocol exists, where it can be accessed, and provide registration information
	Eligibility criteria: Specify study characteristics and report characteristics used as criteria for eligibility, with rationale
	Sources of information: Describe all information sources in the "search" and "date last searched"
	Survey: Present the full electronic search strategy for at least one major database
	Study selection: State the process for selecting studies
	Data collection process: Describe the method of data extraction from reports and processes for obtaining and confirming data
	Data items: List and define all variables for which data were sought and any assumptions made
	Risk of bias in individual studies: Describe methods for assessing the risk of bias in individual studies
	Summary measures: State the principal summary measures (e.g., risk ratio and difference in means)
	Synthesis of outcomes: Explain methods of data use and combination methods of study outcomes
	Risk of bias across studies: Specify any assessment of risk of bias that may affect the cumulative evidence
	Additional analyses: Describe methods of additional analyses, indicating which were prespecified

Continued

Continued

Item	Description
Results	*Study selection:* Give the numbers of studies screened, assessed for eligibility, and included in the review, ideally with a flow diagram
	Study characteristics: For each study, present characteristics and provide the citation
	Risk of bias within studies: Present data on the risk of bias in each study
	Results of individual studies: Present summary data for each intervention group and effect estimates
Discussion	*Summary of evidence:* Summarize the main findings, including the strength of evidence for each main outcome
	Limitations: Discuss limitations at the study, outcome , and review levels
	Conclusions: Provide a general interpretation of the results in the context of other evidence, and implications for future research
Funding	*Funding:* Indicate sources of funding or other support for the systematic review, and the role of funders

This checklist ensures comprehensive and transparent reporting, enhancing the reliability and usefulness of systematic reviews and meta-analyses in health sciences.

This introduction sets the stage for exploring the nuances of writing a review article in the medical field, emphasizing the importance of methodological rigor and clarity in communication to effectively contribute to the advancement of medical science and practice.

Review articles play a crucial role in summarizing and interpreting a vast amount of information in a specific field. Unlike original research, they offer a synthesis of existing studies, providing an overview and critical analysis of a topic. For instance, a review article in medicine might cover the latest treatment strategies for a specific disease, integrating findings from numerous clinical trials and studies to offer a holistic view of the current state of treatment.

SYSTEMATIC VERSUS NONSYSTEMATIC REVIEWS: METHODOLOGIES AND IMPACT ON SCIENTIFIC INTEGRITY

In the realm of scientific literature, the distinction between systematic and nonsystematic reviews is crucial, primarily due to the methodologies employed in sourcing and analyzing literature. Nonsystematic reviews often derive from a collection of articles recommended by peers over the years, while systematic reviews are grounded in a rigorous process of searching for the best possible research to answer predefined questions.

Despite the consensus on the systematic approach for review articles, many fail to adhere to this format. An analysis by McAlister et al. of review articles in six medical journals revealed that less than a quarter provided methods for describing, evaluating, or synthesizing evidence. Only one-third focused on a clinical topic, and merely half offered quantitative data about potential benefits.[7] This highlights a significant gap in the quality of review articles, impacting their reliability and usefulness.

The importance of employing proper methodologies in review articles cannot be overstated. Readers typically approach these articles expecting objective and up-to-date information. However, two primary issues often arise when using data from research to answer specific questions. Firstly, there's the risk of bias in selecting research articles. For instance, a researcher studying the efficacy of a new diabetes medication might unintentionally select studies that show positive outcomes, overlooking those with neutral or negative results. To mitigate this, methodologies in systematic reviews should define and utilize research with minimal bias. Secondly, many research studies suffer from small sample sizes, limiting their statistical power. Meta-analyses in systematic reviews address this by combining multiple studies, thereby enhancing the overall statistical strength.[8] For example, a meta-analysis on the effectiveness of a psychological intervention in treating anxiety could pool results from several small studies, providing a more robust conclusion. In contrast, nonsystematic reviews are susceptible to biased responses. This is because there is a tendency to select studies with familiar or favorable results, rather than choosing based on quality. For example, a nonsystematic review on climate change impacts might lean toward studies that align with the author's viewpoint, ignoring equally relevant but contradictory research.

In summary, while writing a review article, it is imperative to adopt a systematic approach, ensuring the selection of high-quality, unbiased studies. This not only provides a more accurate and comprehensive understanding of the topic but also upholds the integrity and reliability of the review article as a valuable resource in the scientific community.

Table 2 provides a clear and concise format for constructing a systematic review, ensuring comprehensive coverage of the topic and adherence to academic standards.

Table 3 succinctly encapsulates each section's key elements, providing a clear and structured overview of the systematic review process as exemplified by a specific study by Bandyopadhyay et al. on semaglutide's role in treating nonalcoholic fatty liver disease (NAFLD) and nonalcoholic steatohepatitis (NASH), presented in a tabular format.[9]

METHODOLOGICAL FRAMEWORK FOR CRAFTING A SYSTEMATIC REVIEW

In crafting a systematic review, adherence to a structured approach is pivotal for ensuring comprehensiveness and scientific rigor. The systematic review

TABLE 2: Concise format for constructing a systematic review.

Section	Contents
Introduction	Introduces the problem and the issues addressed in the review
	Provides background information and rationale for the review
	States the research questions or objectives
Methods	Details the research process, including data sources and search strategies
	Describes the evaluation process for selecting studies
	Specifies the number of studies evaluated or selected, including inclusion and exclusion criteria
	Explains the methods used for data extraction and any analysis methods (like meta-analysis)
Results	Describes the quality and outcomes of the selected studies
	Presents data in an organized format, often using tables, charts, and, if applicable, forest plots
	Summarizes key findings in a clear and concise manner
Discussion	Summarizes the main results, highlighting significant findings
	Discusses the limitations of the studies included and the review process itself
	Interprets the outcomes in the context of the wider field, discussing implications for practice and research
	Suggests areas for future research based on the review findings

TABLE 3: An example of a systematic review process as exemplified by a specific study.[10]

Section	Contents
Introduction	Highlights the prevalence of NAFLD and NASH and their progression risks
	Introduces semaglutide as a potential treatment
	States the review's purpose: Evaluating semaglutide's efficacy and safety in treating NAFLD/NASH
Methods	Describes the search strategy across databases like PubMed and Scopus
	Specifies inclusion/exclusion criteria (study types, participant characteristics, and intervention details)
	Outlines the process for evaluating study quality and data extraction
Results	Provides a flow diagram of study selection
	Summarizes key data from each study: Sample size, treatment duration, and primary outcomes (e.g., liver fat reduction)
	Details meta-analysis results, if conducted, including statistical methods, effect sizes, and confidence intervals
Discussion	Interprets results in the context of NAFLD and NASH treatment
	Discusses strengths and limitations of the evidence
	Compares semaglutide with other treatments
	Highlights research gaps and suggests future research directions

(NAFLD: nonalcoholic fatty liver disease; NASH: nonalcoholic steatohepatitis)

process involves several key steps that guide researchers from the initial formulation of research questions to the final synthesis of findings:

- *Formulation of researchable questions:* The foundation of a systematic review is to define clear, answerable research questions. For example, in a study by Bandyopadhyay et al., the research question focused on assessing the effects of saroglitazar in treating NAFLD and NASH.[10]
- *Disclosure of studies:* This step involves identifying relevant databases and selecting appropriate keywords for the literature search. In their review on saroglitazar, Bandyopadhyay et al. would have chosen databases like PubMed and used keywords related to NAFLD, NASH, and saroglitazar, ensuring a comprehensive collection of relevant studies.
- *Evaluation of its quality:* A critical part of the process is assessing the quality of selected studies. This includes evaluating study design, methodology, sample size, and potential biases. The quality assessment in the saroglitazar review would have ensured that only studies meeting a certain standard were included in their analysis.
- *Synthesis:* The final step is synthesizing the outcomes of the selected studies, which involves interpreting and combining the results. In the saroglitazar review, this likely involved a meta-analysis to quantitatively combine the results of individual studies, providing a more powerful and comprehensive understanding of saroglitazar's effects.

Each of these steps is crucial for constructing a good review article. The systematic review on saroglitazar by Bandyopadhyay et al. serves as an excellent example, demonstrating the application of these methodological steps in producing a scientifically robust and informative review article in the field of hepatology.[11]

CRAFTING A NARRATIVE REVIEW

Writing a narrative review involves a structured yet flexible approach, distinct from systematic reviews. It typically includes a synthesis or critique of literature on a specific topic, aiming to offer a well-organized, purposeful, and insightful analysis that benefits the reader. The planning phase involves discussions with the journal editor to define the review's purpose, audience, and scope. A thorough literature search is then carried out, and the gathered literature helps to plan the review's structure and outline.

The writing process of a narrative review consists of several key sections:

- *Introduction:* Establishing the rationale for the review is crucial. The introduction should clearly state the review's purpose, flowing logically from the rationale and guiding the rest of the review.
- *Main text:* This section is the core of the narrative review. The foundation of the main text is the writer's own ideas, supported and guided by research. The main text involves summarizing individual studies in the author's own words and paraphrasing statements from studies. It requires skillful synthesis, using transitions to signal similarities, contrasts, or relationships

between studies and interpreting each group of findings as a whole. Additionally, it should identify areas where more research is needed.

- *Conclusion:* The conclusion must correspond to the review's purpose and should be based on the presented material. It often highlights areas where further research is needed.

Example: Considering the paper[12] by Samajdar et al. on "Component-resolved Diagnostics in Allergy Practice Focusing on Food Allergy", the authors would have started with a clear rationale, i.e., understanding the role of component-resolved diagnostics in food allergy practice. The main text would synthesize various studies on this topic, identifying key trends, contrasting different findings, and possibly providing a fresh perspective on the subject. The conclusion would likely reflect on how this approach can shape future allergy practices and pinpoint gaps in current research. In summary, crafting a narrative review involves a well-structured approach, starting from a clear purpose and culminating in a synthesis that not only summarizes existing literature but also provides new insights, offering significant value to the reader.[13]

IMPORTANCE OF PICOT FORMAT

Understanding the PICOT format is integral to formulating a clear and effective research question, especially in the context of exploring the effects of therapeutic interventions. PICOT stands for population, intervention, comparison, outcome, and time.[14]

- *Population (P):* This component refers to the group of subjects under study. Defining the population is crucial for the relevance and applicability of the research. For instance, in a study on arthritis treatment, the population might be "adults aged 50–70 years with osteoarthritis". The aim is to balance specificity (ensuring the sample is representative of those who will receive the intervention) with generalizability (ensuring the findings apply to a broader clinical practice setting).
- *Intervention (I):* This is the treatment or condition being studied. In a review article, clearly describing the intervention allows for a focused analysis. For example, in a review of treatments for hypertension, the intervention might be a specific drug or a lifestyle modification program.
- *Comparison (C):* The comparison typically involves a control group or an alternative treatment. In many studies, this might be the current "gold standard" treatment against which the new intervention is compared. For instance, in a review comparing different surgical techniques for cataract removal, the comparison group could be patients undergoing the traditional surgical method.
- *Outcome (O):* This refers to the results measured to evaluate the intervention's effectiveness. Outcomes should be relevant, measurable,

and clearly defined. In a review article examining a new psychotherapy method for depression, the outcome might be the reduction in depression scores measured by a specific scale like the Beck Depression Inventory.

- *Time (T):* Time specifies the duration of data collection or the time frame over which the outcomes are measured. It is an essential aspect as it impacts the relevance and applicability of the findings. For instance, in a long-term study of a diabetes management program, "time" might refer to patient's follow-up over several years to assess the sustained effects of the intervention.

In summary, the PICOT format provides a structured approach to formulating research questions in a review article. It ensures that the research is targeted, relevant, and methodologically sound, facilitating a more effective synthesis and analysis of the literature in the chosen field of study.

EXPLORING STUDIES

This process should be meticulously planned and clearly detailed in the review article, as it significantly influences the quality and relevance of the findings. When embarking on a systematic review, the methods of investigation, including the databases searched and the keywords used, must be explicitly outlined. The choice of databases is topic dependent; for clinical topics, Medline is often essential. However, databases like Embase and CINAHL might also be relevant, depending on the subject matter. The formulation of search terms is guided by the PICO (population, intervention, comparison, outcome) elements of the research question. In most cases, the population and intervention components are key to defining the search strategy. To ensure a comprehensive search, it is important to consider synonyms for these elements, using logical operators like "AND" to combine them. This approach ensures that the search captures a broad range of relevant studies.

The use of a "methodological filter" can significantly streamline the search process. This approach involves selecting the best investigation method for each research question. A prominent example is the Clinical Queries tool in the PubMed interface of Medline. This tool provides empirically developed filters tailored to specific types of inquiries, such as etiology, diagnosis, treatment, prognosis, or clinical prediction. These filters help researchers quickly identify high-quality studies relevant to their specific research question.[9]

Incorporating these strategies into the search process ensures that the systematic review is grounded in a robust and comprehensive literature search. This methodical approach is essential for the validity and reliability of the review, as it minimizes the risk of missing significant studies and allows for a more accurate representation of the current state of knowledge on the topic.

EVALUATION OF STUDY QUALITY

To write a review article, a critical element is the evaluation of study quality. This involves discerning high-quality research from lesser-quality studies, ensuring that the review's conclusions are based on the most reliable evidence. Understanding the hierarchy of evidence is pivotal in this process as it varies depending on the type of research question and study design. The initial step in quality evaluation is assessing the study's overall design and methodology. This evaluation looks at whether the study is, for instance, a well-structured cohort study, a detailed case series, or a randomized controlled trial. Each of these designs has inherent strengths and limitations that affect the quality and applicability of their findings. A typical hierarchy of evidence categorizes studies based on their methodological rigor and relevance to the research question. This hierarchy serves as a guideline for identifying the most credible and authoritative sources. After pinpointing high-quality studies, the reviewer can focus on these and potentially bypass less-relevant or lower-quality research, saving significant time and effort. In applying this approach, the reviewer undertakes a systematic and critical appraisal of each selected study. This involves looking at various aspects such as the study's sample size, control of variables, statistical analysis, potential biases, and the robustness of the findings. The goal is to ensure that the review article's conclusions are grounded in research that adheres to the highest standards of scientific inquiry. This process of evaluating study quality is not just a procedural step, but it is integral to the integrity and value of the review article itself. By meticulously assessing the quality of the included studies, the reviewer ensures that the synthesis provided is both accurate and representative of the best available evidence in the field.

Table 4 outlines the levels of evidence based on the type of research question, covering areas such as intervention, diagnosis, prognosis, and etiology. This table provides a structured framework for determining the levels of evidence in various research domains, helping researchers and reviewers to assess the strength and reliability of the studies they are reviewing or conducting.

FORMULATING A SYNTHESIS

Formulating a synthesis in a systematic review, especially when studies yield divergent conclusions, requires a nuanced and methodical approach. The process should not rely solely on the majority of studies leaning in a particular direction, as this approach risks giving equal weight to studies of varying qualities. To illustrate this process, let us consider the systematic review and meta-analysis conducted by Joshi et al. on the efficacy and safety of lobeglitazone in type 2 diabetes mellitus.[14] In their review, Joshi et al. likely encountered studies with differing conclusions about lobeglitazone's

TABLE 4: Determination of levels of evidence based on the type of research question.[14]

Level	Intervention	Diagnosis	Prognosis	Etiology
I	Systematic review of Level II studies	Systematic review of Level II studies	Systematic review of Level II studies	Systematic review of Level II studies
II	Randomized controlled study	Cross-sectional study in consecutive patients	Initial cohort study	Prospective cohort study
III	One of the following: • Nonrandomized experimental study (e.g., controlled pre- and post-test intervention study) • Comparative studies with concurrent control groups (observational study) (e.g., cohort study and case–control study)	One of the following: • Cross-sectional study in nonconsecutive case series • Diagnostic case–control study	One of the following: • Untreated control group patients in a randomized controlled study • Integrated cohort study	One of the following: • Retrospective cohort study • Case–control study (Note: these are most prevalently used types of etiological studies; for other alternatives, and interventional studies see Level III)
IV	Case series	Case series	Case series or cohort studies with patients at different stages of their disease states	-

effectiveness and safety. To synthesize these findings effectively, the authors would first focus on the largest and highest-quality study available. This study serves as a benchmark, providing a strong foundation for comparison due to its scale and methodological robustness. Following this, the authors would compare the findings of other studies with this "basic" or benchmark study. This comparison is crucial to understanding how smaller or less-robust studies align or diverge from the findings of the more comprehensive research. For instance, if the benchmark study found lobeglitazone to be highly effective with minimal side effects, but smaller studies reported varied outcomes, these discrepancies would need careful analysis. The meta-analysis part of their review plays a critical role in resolving these apparent differences. Through statistical techniques, the meta-analysis combines data from multiple studies to derive a more precise estimate of lobeglitazone's effects. This process allows for an evaluation that considers both the size and quality of each study, giving more weight to studies with robust design and large sample sizes. The synthesis in the review of Joshi et al. would then present a balanced view, integrating results from the benchmark studies with findings from the meta-analysis. This approach ensures that the review's conclusions are not just a reflection of the majority opinion but are grounded in a rigorous evaluation of the evidence, considering both the quality and quantity of the available research.

In summary, the synthesis in a systematic review should prioritize high-quality studies while using meta-analysis to reconcile differences across research. This method provides a comprehensive and accurate overview of the evidence, as exemplified in Joshi et al.'s review of lobeglitazone in type 2 diabetes mellitus.[15]

CONCLUSION

In conclusion, the journey of writing a review article is both rigorous and enlightening, requiring a meticulous blend of analytical and creative skills.

Key procedures for crafting an effective review article include the following:

- *Embracing an open perspective:* Begin by shedding any preconceived notions or biases. Approach the subject matter with a broad, open-minded perspective. This mindset is crucial for conducting an unbiased and comprehensive review of the literature, ensuring that all relevant aspects of the topic are explored and understood.
- *Methodical and critical research approach:* Dive into the literature with a methodological rigor and a critical eye. This involves systematically searching for studies, carefully evaluating their quality using established criteria, and thoughtfully synthesizing the findings. A critical approach helps in differentiating high-quality research from lesser-quality studies, ensuring that the conclusions drawn are based on the most reliable and relevant evidence.
- *Engaging presentation of data:* Finally, the essence of a well-written review article lies in how the data and findings are conveyed. The synthesis of complex information should not only be accurate and comprehensive but also be presented in an engaging and accessible manner. This involves skillful writing that makes the review both informative and compelling to its audience, regardless of their level of expertise on the subject.

The creation of a review article, therefore, is not just about collating existing knowledge; it is an artful exercise in critical thinking, objective analysis, and creative synthesis. By adhering to these key procedures, the review article becomes a valuable contribution to the academic community, offering insights and understanding that can shape future research and practice in the field.

REFERENCES

1. Oxman AD, Cook DJ, Guyatt GH. Users' guides to the medical literature. VI. How to use an overview. Evidence-Based Medicine Working Group. JAMA. 1994;272(17):1367-71.
2. Mulrow CD. The medical review article: State of the science. Ann Intern Med. 1987;106(3):485-8.
3. Moher D, Cook DJ, Eastwood S, Olkin I, Rennie D, Stroup DF. Improving the quality of reports of meta-analyses of randomised controlled trials: The QUOROM statement. Quality of Reporting of Meta-analyses. Lancet. 1999;354:1896-900.
4. Moher D, Liberati A, Tetzlaff J, Altman DG; PRISMA Group. Preferred reporting items for systematic reviews and meta-analyses: The PRISMA statement. BMJ. 2009;339:b2535.
5. Collins JA, Fauser BC. Balancing the strengths of systematic and narrative reviews. Hum Reprod Update. 2005;11(2):103-4.
6. Booth WC, Colomb GG, Williams JM. The Craft of Research: Chicago Guides to Writing, Editing and Publishing, 2nd edition. Chicago: The University of Chicago Press; 2003.
7. McAlister FA, Clark HD, van Walraven C, Straus SE, Lawson FM, Moher D, et al. The medical review article revisited: Has the science improved? Ann Intern Med. 1999;131:947-51.
8. Gülpınar Ö, Güçlü AG. How to write a review article? Turk J Urol. 2013;39(Suppl 1):44-8.
9. Bandyopadhyay S, Das S, Samajdar SS, Joshi SR. Role of semaglutide in the treatment of nonalcoholic fatty liver disease or non-alcoholic steatohepatitis: A systematic review and meta-analysis. Diabetes Metab Syndr. 2023;17(10):102849.
10. Bandyopadhyay S, Samajdar SS, Das S. Effects of saroglitazar in the treatment of non-alcoholic fatty liver disease or non-alcoholic steatohepatitis: A systematic review and meta-analysis. Clin Res Hepatol Gastroenterol. 2023;47(7):102174.
11. Samajdar SS, Mukherjee S, Ghosh S, Munshi S, Tripathi SK, Moitra S, et al. Component-resolved Diagnostics in Allergy Practice Focusing on Food Allergy: A Systematic Review. Bengal Physician Journal. 2023;10(2):29-42.
12. Riva JJ, Malik KM, Burnie SJ, Endicott AR, Busse JW. What is your research question? An introduction to the PICOT format for clinicians. J Can Chiropr Assoc. 2012;56(3):167-71.
13. Glasziou PP, Vandenbroucke J, Chalmers I. Assessing the quality of research. BMJ. 2004;328:39-41.
14. Joshi SR, Das S, Xaviar S, Samajdar SS, Saha I, Sarkar S, et al. Efficacy and safety of lobeglitazone, a new Thiazolidinedione, as compared to the standard of care in type 2 diabetes mellitus: A systematic review and meta-analysis. Diabetes Metab Syndr. 2023; 17(1):102703.

CHAPTER 7

Clinical Images: Spot the Diagnosis

Atanu Chandra

INTRODUCTION

Clinical images possess the power to convey medical scenarios vividly and succinctly. For novice authors, navigating the landscape of clinical image publications can be both exciting and challenging. Clinical images serve as visual aids that enhance medical literature's educational and clinical values. They provide a tangible representation of rare conditions, diagnostic challenges, and treatment outcomes, enriching the reader's understanding of medical concepts. Image-based medical articles play a pivotal role in disseminating research findings and advancing medical knowledge. However, the journey from preparing an article to its successful publication involves multiple crucial steps.

BASICS OF PREPARATION OF CLINICAL IMAGE-BASED ARTICLES

Image-based medical publications play a crucial role in advancing scientific knowledge and disseminating critical information within the medical community.[1] These articles combine visual representations with informative text, allowing researchers, clinicians, and scholars to communicate findings effectively.

What type of images are suitable for publication?: Clinical photographs, radiological images [X-rays, computed tomography (CT) scans, magnetic resonance imaging (MRI)], histological and cytological images, and step-by-step images of medical procedures

How to prepare an image-based article?: Organize your article in a logical flow. Ensure images are high resolution and well lit. Write informative captions that explain the significance of each image. Provide a thorough analysis of the images, including context, findings, and clinical implications.

How to select journals suitable for publication?: Choose journals that align with the subject matter of your images and research. Consider journals with a reputable impact factor in the field. Familiarize yourself with the specific requirements and guidelines of your target journals.

Difficulties in publishing image-based articles: Poor-quality images can hinder understanding and impact the chances of publication. Nonadherence to patient confidentiality and ethical guidelines, when sharing images, increases the chances of rejection. Ensure accurate interpretation of images to avoid misrepresentation.

Strategies to overcome challenges: Work with experts in medical imaging to ensure image quality and interpretation. Obtain necessary permissions and ethical approvals before using patient images. Seek feedback from colleagues to refine both textual and visual content.

PREPARATION OF AN IMAGE-BASED ARTICLE

Capturing impactful images requires meticulous preparation and adherence to guidelines. The first step of preparation of an image-based article is to study the specific guidelines of the target journal meticulously to understand the preferred image format, resolution, and other requirements. Select an image that conveys a clear and intriguing medical scenario, highlighting a relevant clinical condition or treatment outcome. Ensure that patient's consent and privacy standards are met before using any patient-related images. Images that showcase rare conditions, unique presentations, diagnostic challenges, treatment outcomes, and educational value are ideal for this section. Clinical photographs, radiological images, endoscopic visuals, and histopathology slides are often included. The preparation of the manuscript also needs adherence to some checklists. Craft a concise but informative title. Cryptic titles should better be avoided. The manuscript text should include essential details about the patient, clinical context, and key findings. The sequence should be in the following order: History of the patient, clinical examination findings, investigation details, treatment provided, outcome/follow-up, differential diagnosis, how diagnosis is reached, and lastly a brief discussion on the condition including its importance.

QUALITIES OF A GOOD CLINICAL IMAGE FOR PUBLICATION

A good-quality clinical image is not merely a snapshot but a canvas that captures medical narratives vividly. By adhering to the following qualities, authors can enhance their chances of publication of a clinical image in an esteemed journal:

- Ensure high-resolution images with clear focus and proper lighting. The image should be free from artifacts, blurriness, or distortions. Adequate

illumination ensures clarity and accurate representation of colors and textures, fostering accurate interpretation.
- Ethical standards demand that the patient's identity remains protected, with no identifying features or information visible in the image.
- A neutral, uncluttered background eliminates distractions and keeps the focus on the clinical subject.
- Maintain consistency in image quality, framing, and patient positioning. This enhances visual comprehension and comparability. Refrain from using accessories or ornaments when photographing areas like the neck or hands, as these could detract from the clinical context.
- An image should not be too shocking, disturbing, or graphic. It should strike a balance between conveying information and respecting the sensitivity of the audience.
- While not overly common, the image should also avoid being too rare. Classic presentations of clinical conditions tend to resonate well with audiences.
- High-resolution images with sharp focus capture nuances and details crucial for accurate interpretation.
- In case of publishing radiological images (X-rays, CT, or MRI), try to collect soft copies of the relevant images. It is not preferable to put the image in the view box and click an image. Always keep the follow-up images as backup, as most of the reputed journals ask to submit the follow-up images during revision.

JOURNEY FROM PREPARATION TO PUBLICATION

The journey from preparing an image-based medical article to its successful publication involves careful planning and resilience. Selecting the right journal, adhering to guidelines, and addressing feedback are crucial steps. Rejections are a part of the process, but with determination, improvement continues, and researchers can enhance their chances of successful publication and contribute significantly to the medical field's advancement.

Following are some of the important factors that should be kept in mind:
- Selecting the right journal is a critical step. Factors such as the journal's impact factor, scope, readership, and indexation in reputable databases like PubMed should be considered. Additionally, assessing publication charges, open-access options, and the journal's reputation within the field can guide your decision.
- To minimize the chances of rejection, ensure that your article aligns with the journal's scope and formatting guidelines. Thoroughly proofread for language and grammar errors. Highlight the novelty and significance of your findings. Address ethical considerations and disclose conflicts of interest and funding sources transparently.

- Images for the article should be of optimum quality (already discussed earlier).
- Rejection is common in the publication process. Take rejection as an opportunity to learn and improve. Carefully review the reviewer's comments and editor's feedback. If the feedback is constructive, consider revising the article and submitting it to a different journal. Persistence is the key.
- If your article faces repeated rejections, re-evaluate your research and its presentation. Seek feedback from colleagues and mentors. Consider revising the article, restructuring it, or even conducting further experiments to strengthen your findings. Exploring different journals with varying scopes might also be beneficial.

REJECTION FROM ONE JOURNAL: WHY AND WHAT TO DO NEXT?

Common factors that lead to rejection include the following:

- *Insufficient quality:* Poor image resolution, blurriness, or inadequate lighting can lead to rejection.
- *Lack of context:* Images without comprehensive clinical information or context might fail to convey the medical significance effectively.
- *Ethical concerns:* Inadequate patient consent or privacy issues can lead to immediate rejection.
- *Lack of novelty:* Images that are too common and nonspecific for a clinical condition, and if the article does not add much to the existing literature, have lesser chances of acceptance.

If rejected from one journal, if possible, analyze the feedback provided by the journal. It may offer insights into the reasons for rejection. Address the concerns raised and revise the images and manuscript accordingly. Then, consider submitting to another suitable journal.

REAL-LIFE EXAMPLES FROM THE AUTHOR

The author has image-based publications in numerous peer-reviewed indexed journals including the *New England Journal of Medicine* (*NEJM*), the Lancet, Quarterly Journal of Medicine (QJM), American Journal of Medicine, British Medical Journal (BMJ) Case Reports, and several dermatology journals. I would like to tell the readers about our publication stories in the NEJM and the Lancet. A patient presented to us in the outpatients department with the complaint of night blindness and my junior colleague discovered Bitot's spots on ocular examination. Photographs were taken with a mobile camera. We prepared the manuscript and submitted it to the NEJM. But unfortunately, it was rejected. On the very next day, we submitted it to the Lancet. After 2 weeks, we got an email from the editorial team that the article would be accepted after some minor revisions.[2]

During the coronavirus disease (COVID) pandemic, one male patient was admitted to our institution with features suggestive of chronic liver disease. On examination of the eyes, I suddenly found the classical Kayser-Fleischer (K–F) rings visible to the naked eyes. Further evaluations proved the diagnosis of Wilson's disease. But the slit lamp was out of order in our institution then. To click a good-quality photograph, we sent the patient to the regional center of ophthalmology, Kolkata; the transport was arranged by us and the patient was accompanied by one responsible junior resident. After getting the photographs, I could not believe my own eyes as they were of excellent quality. We submitted them to the NEJM, and we got a positive email from their side after 3 months. The article got accepted after a few minor revisions.[3]

My second publication in the NEJM was a clinical photograph of a patient with chronic arsenicosis. The middle-aged female patient presented to us with the complaint of gradual darkening of the skin. The hyperkeratosis of the palm/soles and the "rain-drop pigmentation" were classical. She was admitted under our care. We did the relevant investigations, and she was sent to a nearby institution for the quantitative estimation of arsenic from her nails and hairs. Again, the transport was arranged by us, and the patient was accompanied by one responsible junior resident. After getting the reports, we submitted the case report to the NEJM and got a positive response from the editorial board after 2 months. Subsequently, the article got published after 5 months of submission.[4]

ROLE OF ARTIFICIAL INTELLIGENCE AND CHATGPT IN PREPARATION OF IMAGE-BASED ARTICLES

The field of clinical medicine is evolving, and so are the tools available to medical professionals and researchers. Artificial intelligence (AI), particularly ChatGPT, has started to play a significant role in the preparation of image spotter-type articles. AI tools like ChatGPT can assist in drafting different sections of an article by generating coherent and contextually relevant text. AI also aids in refining the language, grammar, and style of the article, ensuring its readability and professionalism. It can assist in managing citations and references, ensuring accuracy and proper formatting. AI can provide suggestions for relevant images, graphs, and figures to complement the text, enhancing the overall presentation. ChatGPT accelerates the writing process, leaving researchers with more time to focus on the analysis and interpretation of findings. It also ensures consistent language usage and adherence to formatting guidelines throughout the article. AI can be especially helpful for non-native English speakers, improving the overall quality of language.

On the other hand, AI may sometimes misinterpret medical jargon or fail to capture the nuances required in clinical descriptions. Over-reliance on AI can result in content that lacks the researcher's personal touch and unique insights. AI-generated content might miss out on critical clinical nuances, requiring human verification and refinement. Always use AI to draft initial sections, but ensure thorough review and editing to retain the article's accuracy and authenticity. Employ AI for grammar and style checks, but rely on medical professionals for context-specific review. AI-generated suggestions for images can be valuable, but the final decision should rest with the author, considering the clinical relevance.

CONCLUSION

The most important step in the publication of a clinical image-based article is to have an idea whether the image is publishable or not (e.g., an interesting image of tuberculosis has a high chance of acceptance in any European journal but a high chance of rejection in any Indian journal). This needs considerable knowledge about the basics of publication of such articles; the beginners should take advice from colleagues who are much more efficient in publishing. Image-based medical publications provide a powerful platform to share insights, advancements, and discoveries in the field of medicine. By carefully selecting and preparing images, adhering to ethical considerations, and overcoming potential challenges, researchers and clinicians can effectively contribute to the scientific community. Through collaboration, attention to detail, and adherence to guidelines, image-based articles can drive progress in medical knowledge and patient care.

- The most important step in the publication of a clinical image-based article is to have an idea of whether the image is publishable or not.
- Images for the article should be of optimum quality.
- If rejected from one journal, if possible, analyze the feedback provided by the journal. It may offer insights into the reasons for rejection. Address the concerns raised and revise the image and manuscript accordingly. Then, consider submitting to another suitable journal.

REFERENCES

1. Jambor H, Antonietti A, Alicea B, Audisio TL, Auer S, Bhardwaj V, et al. Creating clear and informative image-based figures for scientific publications. PLoS Biol. 2021;19(3):e3001161.
2. Chakraborty U, Chandra A. Bitot's spots, dry eyes, and night blindness indicate vitamin A deficiency. Lancet. 2021;397(10270):e2.
3. Chandra A, Bhattacharjee MS. Kayser–Fleischer Rings in Wilson's Disease. N Engl J Med. 2021;385(14):e46.
4. Chandra A, Shah KA. Chronic Arsenic Poisoning. N Engl J Med. 2022;387(15):1414.

CHAPTER 8

Letter to the Editor

Arnab Bhattacharyya

INTRODUCTION

The section "letter to the editor" is an essential part of a scientific journal, where a short form of communication is established between the reader and the author, with the editor as its mediator. Even though every article is meticulously scrutinized before its publication in a peer-reviewed scientific journal, errors do happen, and in that scenario, "letter to the editor" is there to keep a strict vigil on the quality of the scientific publication, as it expresses the reader's comments about a particular article, and thus the quality control mechanism still proceeds even after publication of the article in a peer-reviewed scientific journal. It may otherwise be stated that any kind of publication is just the beginning of a new process or (so as to say) a scientific dialogue where the reader and the author of an article can interact.

HOW TO WRITE A LETTER TO THE EDITOR OR WHAT ARE ITS SPECIAL CHARACTERISTICS?

Although the most frequent reason for writing a letter to the editor is to communicate a comment (i.e., complementing or criticizing) about a previously published article, letters may also be written for the purpose of communicating scientific discourse in a brief manner. Thus, research reports, case series, or an adverse reaction to a drug can also be reported as a letter. In fact, letters can be written on every important topic that attracts the attention of the readers. And for this purpose, the letters must be published under the surveillance of the editor, as the contents of the letter must be verified before its publication. The language must be very courteous and polite, and there should not be any ostentatious claim about the scientific basis of a research or case series. Even while criticizing an article instead of using rude, pedantic, or pejorative expressions, a professional and elegant approach should be followed. The letter should have some objectives and every information should be constructive, unbiased, and based on scientific evidence (references to previous relevant important literature should be noted). Here comes the role of an editor. He is there to scrutinize the authenticity of the information and to check the clarity of the arguments (for or against the topic) raised by the reader (toward the author) so as to protect the reputation of the researcher and not to discredit the researcher unnecessarily.

The communication must be bidirectional. There should be a way by which an author may be able to respond to questions (arguments) raised by the reader, thus increasing the clarity of the information supplied by the author or the reader. This interaction between the readers and authors of a journal creates a scientific dialogue or debate, which actually favors the impact factor of the journal by increasing the number of citations of a published article (being criticized or analyzed), thereby increasing the journal's rate of acceptance. But in all respects the letter must be brief and concise as the editors of scientific journals like short communications (usually 200–500 words or as set by journal's format) in this section, so that they can accommodate quite a few comments from different readers about the same topic (preferably different topics) within a short space. Moreover, a short and comprehensive communication will deliver information more readily than a long and tedious scientific discourse.

Again, this section of a scientific journal has got some pedagogical values also, as it helps new researchers to get acquainted with the process of publication under the surveillance of an editor, as well as help them to familiarize themselves with constructive, evidence-based, scientific criticism. In this respect, it is worth mentioning that the International Committee of Medical Journal Editors (ICMJE) recommends the publication of these letters along with their responses.[1] Some MEDLINE index journals treat these letters with the responses as original articles just to add extra importance to this valuable section of the journal.[2]

TYPES OF LETTERS

There may be two types of letters:[3] (1) Common type, pertaining to comment on the previously published article or a short but comprehensive feedback on clinical data, research data, or case reports, and (2) Uncommon type, which deals with common medical issues or journal's policy, quality, or format. There may also be comments regarding study materials. Often, letters may refer to a new hypothesis or may report a new experimental result (these observations often may not meet the criteria for the original article on account of their length and importance). There may be caveats regarding the use of a new drug or lifestyle modification of patients or any medicolegal issue.

While commenting on a previously published article or expressing thoughts relating to new insights regarding the hypothesis, case series, or novel effects of a drug, a title may be added to the article.[4] A "Title", if added, should be short, relevant, and at the same time eye-catching.

Some examples of letters that showcase these variations are as follows:

- *Common type*:
  - "Revisiting screening for autonomic neuropathy":[5] In this letter, the writer has congratulated the authors of the article.
  - "Necessity of baseline diabetic autonomic neuropathy screening to start cardiovascular safety outcome trials: A focus on antidiabetic agents and autonomic neurointegrity"[6] for discussing such an important issue in an elaborate manner. Here, the writer has expressed some positive comments in favor of the authors.
- *Uncommon type:*
  - "Hit the iron when it is red hot"[7]: In this letter, the writer has nurtured a new idea that the adult vaccination program in a large country like India (with more than 90 crores adult population[7]) may be boosted by the effects of mass vaccination against COVID-19 (coronavirus disease-2019), as this has probably increased the awareness and acceptability of vaccination among Indian adults.

(Readers are advised to go through the full texts of these letters through the links provided in the respective references.)

CONCLUSION

The section "letter to the editor" is an integral part of any journal, and as such the discussion in this section should be authentic, unbiased, and based on scientific evidence. The language needs to be lucid and polite. Writers of such letters should refrain from sending ambiguous messages and instead, they should always endeavor to deliver an understandable message in a very concise manner. The implementation of a maximum word limit is imperative, as mandated by the respective scientific journal.

As the information, delivered in the section letter to the editor should be short and comprehensive (with constructive comments on a published article or an idea regarding a recent scientific discourse), the subject must be well studied before such letters are written.

REFERENCES

1. Uniform requirements for manuscripts submitted to biomedical journals: Writing and editing for biomedical publication. J Pharmacol Pharmacother. 2010;1(1):42-58.
2. Winker MA, Fontanarosa PB. Letters: A forum for scientific discourse. JAMA. 1999;281(16):1543.
3. Süer E, Yaman Ö. How to write an editorial letter? Turk J Urol. 2013;39(Suppl 1):41-3.

4. Castro-Rodríguez Y. (2021). The letter to the editor in scientific publications: Considerations for its preparations. [online] Available from https://www.odon.edu.uy/ojs/index.php/ode/article/view/341 [Last accessed January, 2024].
5. Bhattacharyya A. Revisiting Screening for Autonomic Neuropathy. Bengal Physician Journal 2022;9(2):58.
6. Samajdar SS, Mukherjee S, Joshi S, Tripathi SK. Necessity of Baseline Diabetic Autonomic Neuropathy Screening to Start Cardiovascular Safety Outcome Trials: A Focus on Antidiabetic Agents and Autonomic Neurointegrity. Bengal Physician Journal 2022;9(1):9-12.
7. Bhattacharyya A, De N, Sarkar S, De SC. Hit the Iron When it is Red Hot. Bengal Physician Journal 2023;10(1):26.

CHAPTER 9

Citation Principles

Nandini Chatterjee

INTRODUCTION

Any publication requires insightful analysis of data and findings compared with that of other studies or reports. This entails referring to multiple external sources or previous documentation. Publication ethics mandate that each source of information be given due credit and that too following certain guidelines.

Citation is a standardized method of acknowledging sources of information and ideas used in a publication. It also helps to identify the source. Direct quotations, facts, figures, as well as ideas and theories, are referenced.[1]

WHY DO WE NEED TO CITE?

- To acknowledge others' work
- To support an argument
- To differentiate other authors' work from one's own results
- To help locate sources of information
- To improve the credibility of own work
- To assess the uniqueness and scope of the manuscripts
- To avoid plagiarism by using the proper citation

WHAT TYPE OF SOURCES SHOULD BE CITED?

- Original, peer-reviewed journal articles, and primary research articles penned by the participants of the studies should be cited.
- Review papers, or secondary sources, can be used in the absence of primary sources.
- The most pertinent, reliable, and methodologically sound papers ought to be chosen.

- The most recent publications ought to be chosen, since they probably discuss and make reference to earlier research.

WHAT ARE THE STYLES OF CITATION?

- The Vancouver system of consecutive numbering
- The well-known Harvard author name–publication year system
- Other systems prescribed by individual journals such as the American Psychological Association (APA), Chicago Manual of Style, Modern Languages Association (MLA), and Modern Humanities Research Association (MHRA).

However, it should be kept in mind that various disciplines have different norms and conventions and may follow different styles of citation.[2]

WHAT ARE THE COMPONENTS OF CITATION?[3]

- Quoting from others, directly or indirectly
- In-text citation
- Bibliographic information of the source

Quoting from Others

- *Direct quotations:* In direct quotations, the exact words (more than six consecutive words) must be put down within quotation marks. This should be followed by an in-text citation to the original source.

  They are used to communicate well-known facts or to furnish background information on a specific theory. In the UK style, one uses "single" quotation marks, while in the US style, one uses "double" quotation marks.
- *Paraphrasing*: Here the authors express other people's views in their own words followed by a reference to the original source.
- *Summary:* A concise statement of the principal findings of a study is presented, and at times the authors present their own viewpoints and opinions too (affiliating or distancing).

In-text Citations

The in-text citations are consecutive numbers in the Vancouver style. They are put either in superscript or within brackets (according to journal instructions) after a full stop/comma. A sentence's middle may contain an in-text reference. Clubbing all of the references at the end of a sentence is not desirable. However, if a text contains multiple references at a single location, a hyphen should be used to join the first and last inclusive numbers, like 6-8.

Commas (with no spaces) are used to separate noninclusive numbers, e.g., 5,7,9. Multiple references should be cited in a chronological order.

In the Harvard style, in-text citation within the text mentions the author's name and date of publication.

Compilation

Reference list: Entries may be listed numerically in the order of "in-text citation" as in the Vancouver style.

The reference list is a detailed list of all the sources cited including books, e-books, journal articles, theses, webpages, etc.

At times, the entries may be listed alphabetically, called the bibliography. This is done in the Harvard style. A bibliography is a compilation of all the works that were used in manuscript preparation but that were not necessarily referred to.

WHAT DO WE NEED TO KNOW ABOUT REFERENCING STYLES?

The Vancouver and Harvard styles are the most common styles to be followed by medical publications. There are many versions of the Harvard and Vancouver referencing styles, but we need to follow the rules established by the International Committee of Medical Journal Editors **(Box 1)**.

Vancouver Style[4]

Vancouver is a "numbered" style with consecutive in-text numbering that matches the corresponding references at the end of the article in the reference list. Only the first letters of the article title and words that begin with a capital letter are capitalized. Journal titles are abbreviated. A list of abbreviations for the titles is available online at the National Library of Medicine (NLM) catalog: Journal abbreviation.

Author(s)/editor(s)/organization's name [Internet]. Title of the article. Place of publication: Publisher's name; [updated year month day; cited year month day]. Available from: URL.

Harvard Style[5]

An in-text citation is added within the text mentioning the author's name and date of publication each time the source is referred to. Compilation is done in an alphabetical order according to the first author's surname.

It is to be noted that the order in which in-text citations appear within the article will not match the reference list; alphabetical arrangement by author/ editor will be done.

Author(s) name, initial(s). (year of publication) Title of article, Title of Journal, volume (issue number), [or] (date/month of publication) [in the absence of volume and issue], page number(s).

BOX 1 Examples of citation styles.

Examples of Vancouver Style

- *Print journal article*
  - Authors less than 6:

    Halpern SD, Ubel PA, Caplan AL. Solid-organ transplantation in HIV-infected patients. N Engl J Med. 2002;347(4):284-7.
  - Authors more than 6:

    Rose ME, Huerbin MB, Melick J, Marion DW, Palmer AM, Schiding JK, et al. Regulation of interstitial excitatory amino acid concentrations after cortical contusion injury. Brain Res. 2002;935(1-2):40-6.
- *Online-only journal article:* Dark P, Dunn G, Chadwick P. The clinical diagnostic accuracy of rapid detection of healthcare-associated bloodstream infection in intensive care using multipathogen real-time PCR technology. BMJ Open. 2011;1:e000181. doi: 10.1136/bmjopen-2011-000181
- *Book reference*
  - Less than 6 editors:

    Murray PR, Rosenthal KS, Kobayashi GS, Pfaller MA. Medical microbiology. 4th ed. St. Louis: Mosby; 2002.
  - More than 6 editors:

    Fauci AS, Braunwald E, Isselbacher KJ, Wilson JD, Martin JB, Kasper DL, et al, editors. Harrison's principles of internal medicine. 14th ed. New York: McGraw Hill; 1998.

Examples of Harvard Style

- *Print journal source*:

  Fisher, E. (2018) Law and energy transitions: wind turbines and planning law in the UK, Oxford Journal of Legal Studies, 38(3), pp. 528-56.
- *Internet source*:

  Jones, P. (2021) Are winters in Ireland getting colder? Irish Energy Blog, 7 February. Available at: http://irishenergyblog.blogspot.com/2021/02/are-winters-in-ireland-getting-colder.html (Accessed: 19 April 2021).

E-BOOKS

The reference list entry for an e-book includes the author, date, title, and source [URL or digital object identifier (DOI)]. For a chapter in an e-book, the chapter title and page numbers (if available) are included. The in-text citation includes the number or author and date, according to the style used.

WHAT ARE FURTHER READINGS?

Sometimes, an article, especially in books, may be followed by a list of sources with the heading "Further Readings".

Further readings allude to sources that the author feels should be consulted by the reader for additional information. However, there are no in-text citations.

HOW MANY REFERENCES SHOULD BE ADDED?

The numbers vary from journal to journal. On an average,

- *Case report*:10–15
- *Pictorial CME*: 4–5
- *Review*: 50–100 (may go over 100 in systematic reviews)

However, it should be borne in mind that referencing should be optimal. Too few may look under-researched, while too much will seem repetitive and redundant.

WHAT ARE THE AVAILABLE HELP IN DIGITAL MODE?[6]

In-text references can be readily connected to the reference list using citation management software (e.g., Mendeley, EndNote, Reference Manager, RefWorks, ProCite, and refbase). These programs have the ability to format bibliographic information and in-text references in a variety of styles and between different styles.

CAN INTERNET SOURCES BE CITED?

They are cited just like their printed counterparts in Vancouver or Harvard styles. The URL and DOI are terms in use.

URL stands for Uniform Resource Locator. A URL is the address of a given unique resource on the Web/Web page.

An article or document can be permanently identified and linked to on the internet with the use of a DOI, which is a string of numbers, letters, and symbols. A DOI makes it simple for readers to find a document from the citation.

Webpage citation:
Author, A. [if no author, use source] (Year, Date). Title. Website name [if used as author, do not repeat website name/source]. URL

Example: Avramova, N. (2019, January 3). The secret of a long, happy, healthy life? Think age-positive. CNN. https://www.cnn.com/2019/01/03/health/respect-toward-elderly-leads-to-a-long-life-intl/index.html

WHAT IS TO BE KNOWN ABOUT CITATION ERRORS?

Citation errors, such as incorrect quotations and reference list errors, are prevalent in medical publications. Between 10 and 20% of journal articles contain misquotations, and between 50 and 70% of reference lists have at least one error.[7]

Inaccurate quotations not only disrespect the cited author but also mislead the reader. They entail circulation of false facts, difficulty in reference retrieval, and faults in citation indexes.

WHAT IS SELF-CITATION?[8]

Self-citation is defined as citing one's own past studies in an article. It helps to strengthen one's findings as a continuum of previous work. However, both irrelevant self-citation and excessive self-citation are unethical and affect the credibility of the paper.

WHAT TO AVOID WHILE CITING SOURCES?

- Incorrect quotation marks and misplaced references are two common citation errors found in medical publications.
- 10–20% of journal articles have misquoted passages, and 50–70% of reference lists have one or more errors.
- Other documents that are not found in the public domain like theses, conference proceeding papers, unpublished data, abstracts, and personal communications are not recommended to be cited unless they contain essential information not available from public sources.
- Standard textbooks are not cited except for enumerating a methodologic principle or a statistical procedure.
- The references cited should not be retracted articles.

Inaccurate citations consist of instances of multiple similar references to support a single statement or using a single source to support multiple statements. It is important to go through the full text of an article to comprehend it and then cite it.

HOW IS THE IMPACT FACTOR OF A JOURNAL RELATED TO CITATION?

The impact factor (IF) is a measure of the frequency with which any article in a journal has been cited in a particular year. It is used to measure the importance or rank of a journal by calculating the times its articles are cited.[9]

Calculation of 2023 IF of a journal:[10]

A = The number of times articles published in 2021 and 2022 were cited by indexed journals during 2023

B = The total number of "citable items" published in 2021 and 2023

A/B = 2023 IF

The IF is reported in Journal Citation Reports (JCR).

WHAT IS THE *h*-INDEX?

The *h*-index measures a researcher's or scientist's performance based on his or her research publications and lifetime citations. The IF evaluates the journal and *h*-index evaluates the author. For example, *h*-index of an author is 31 if 31 articles have each received at least 31 citations. The *h*-index measurement is based on the quantity of publications and number of citations of the author concerned.

CONCLUSION

A well-cited manuscript establishes the credibility of a study and amplifies the reputation of the author. The most valid and recent sources should be selected for citation. Moreover, care should be taken to provide details in the reference list that are accurate and complete to ensure that readers will be able to locate the documents readily.

Most importantly, giving credit by citation avoids plagiarism and copyright infringements as well. Thus, it is imperative to learn citation principles thoroughly when we embark on manuscript writing.

REFERENCES

1. University Libraries, University of Washington. (2023). Citing Sources: What are citations and why should I use them? [online] Available from https://guides.lib.uw.edu/research/citations/citationwhat [Last accessed January, 2024].
2. Penders B. Ten simple rules for responsible referencing. PLoS Comput Biol. 2018;14(4):e1006036.
3. The University of Mississippi Medical Center. (2023). Citation Format: ICMJE/NLM Style. [online] Available from https://umc.libguides.com/citations/nlm. [Last accessed January, 2024].
4. The University of Sydney. (2024). Library, Referencing and Citation Styles: About Vancouver referencing. [online] Available from https://libguides.library.usyd.edu.au/c.php?g=508212&p=3476168 [Last accessed January, 2024].
5. The Open University. (2024). Quick guide to Harvard referencing (Cite Them Right). [online] Available from https://www5.open.ac.uk/library/referencing-and-plagiarism/quick-guide-to-harvard-referencing-cite-them-right [Last accessed January, 2024].
6. Patrias K. In: Wendling DL (Ed). Citing Medicine: The NLM Style Guide for Authors, Editors, and Publishers, 2nd edition. Bethesda (MD): National Library of Medicine; 2007.
7. Ghai B, Saxena AK, Makkar JK. A guide to reducing citation errors in bibliographies. Emerg Med J. 2007;24(3):232-3.
8. Hyland K. Self-citation and self-reference: Credibility and promotion in academic publication. Journal of the Association for Information Science and Technology. 2003;54(3):251-9.
9. Esposito M. The impact factor: Its use, misuse, and significance. Eur J Oral Implantol. 2009;2(2):87.
10. Garfield E. The history and meaning of the journal impact factor. JAMA. 2006;295(1):90-3.

CHAPTER 10

Overview of Guidelines for Publication

Avijit Hazra

INTRODUCTION

Publication is an indispensable component of scientific work. Researchers need to present their scientific findings in order to communicate new knowledge to the community in general, improve their standing in the scientific community, and improve career prospects. Physicians and other healthcare providers need to read and understand scientific work in order to stay up to date in their knowledge and apply the same appropriately in their professional practice. Therefore, it helps if there are universally acceptable guidelines for reporting various types of scientific work, which will facilitate both publication and consumption of scientific literature. In this chapter, we will take an overview of the current scenario with regard to publication guidelines.

Way back in 1978, the International Committee of Medical Journal Editors (ICMJE) first notified a document named Uniform Requirements for Manuscripts Submitted to Biomedical Journals. Over the years various issues beyond simple submission, peer review, and publication arose to address which guidelines have been periodically revised and updated. Currently, the guidelines are called Recommendations for the Conduct, Reporting, Editing, and Publication of Scholarly Work in Medical Journals and were last updated in January 2024. All ICMJE member journals follow these criteria, and many other journals also voluntarily accept these recommendations. The salient features of the current version of the guidelines are provided in **Box 1**.

A perusal of the list in **Box 1** indicates the range and depth of issues that are covered by these guidelines. Some of the items are extremely important and, if followed, can solve many contentious issues. They are highlighted in the following sections.

BOX 1 Salient issues covered by ICMJE Recommendations for the Conduct, Reporting, Editing, and Publication of Scholarly Work in Medical Journals.[1]

The roles and responsibilities of authors, contributors, reviewers, editors, publishers, and owners are as follows:

- Defining the role of authors and contributors:
  - Why authorship matters?
  - Authorship criteria
  - Nonauthor contributors
  - Artificial intelligence (AI)-assisted technology
- Disclosure of financial and nonfinancial relationships and activities, and conflicts of interest covering participants, authors, peer reviewers, editors, and journal staff
- Responsibilities in the submission and peer-review process:
  - Author responsibilities with respect to proper journal selection
  - Journal responsibilities with respect to confidentiality, timeliness, peer review, integrity, diversity and inclusion, and journal metrics
  - Peer reviewer responsibilities
- Journal owners and editorial freedom
- Protection of research participants

Publishing and editorial issues related to publication in medical journals:

- Corrections, retractions, republications, and version control
- Scientific misconduct, expressions of concern, and retraction
- Copyright
- Overlapping publications:
  - Duplicate submission
  - Duplicate and prior publication
  - Preprints
  - Acceptable secondary publication
  - Manuscripts based on the same database
- Correspondence
- Fees
- Supplements, theme issues, and special series
- Sponsorship or partnerships
- Electronic publishing
- Advertising
- Journals and the media
- *Clinical trials:* Registration and Data sharing

Manuscript preparation and submission:

- Preparing a manuscript for submission to a medical journal
  - General principles
  - Reporting guidelines
  - *Manuscript sections:* Title page, abstract, introduction, methods (selection and description of participants, technical information, and statistics), results, discussion, references (general considerations, style, and format), tables, illustrations (figures), units of measurement, abbreviations, and symbols
- Sending the manuscript to the journal

AUTHORSHIP CRITERIA[2]

The ICMJE recommends that only individuals who have actively contributed to the work and fulfill all four of the following criteria be considered as authors:

1. Substantial contributions to the conception or design of the work, or the acquisition, analysis, or interpretation of data, *and*
2. Drafting the work or revising it critically for important intellectual content, *and*
3. Final approval of the version to be published, *and*
4. Agreeing to be accountable for all aspects of the work in ensuring that questions related to the accuracy or integrity of any part of the work are appropriately investigated and resolved.

In addition to being accountable for the part of the work one has done, an author should be able to identify which coauthors are responsible for other parts of the work. In addition, authors should have confidence in the integrity of the contributions from their coauthors. The corresponding author has special responsibility of communication with the journal during the manuscript submission, peer review, and publication process and must also ensure that all the journal's administrative requirements, such as providing details of authors' contributions, ethics committee approval, clinical trial registration, disclosures of relationships, and conflicts of interest, are properly addressed. Individuals who have in some way contributed to the work but do not satisfy all four criteria of authorship may be acknowledged as nonauthor contributors.

When a large multiauthor group has conducted the work, the group leaders should decide who will be the author before the work is started and confirm the sequence of authorship at the time of manuscript submission. All members named as authors should meet all four criteria for authorship, including approval of the final manuscript, and they should be willing to take public responsibility for the work and should have full confidence in the integrity of the work of other group members.

PROTECTION OF PARTICIPANTS IN CLINICAL RESEARCH[3]

Research involving human participants brings along many ethical issues and dilemmas. Today, there is a general consensus that all clinical research must proceed with three ethical safeguards:

1. Conformation to the declaration of Helsinki. The original 1964 declaration has undergone many revisions, and the last major one was the 2013 Fortaleza revision. It is currently under further revision.
2. Research oversight needs to be provided by an appropriately constituted institutional Ethics Committee or Institutional Review Board, which reviews the study protocol, approves the study, and oversees the conduct of the same. Where needed, oversight is also to be provided by a scientific review board.

3. Written informed consent is required from each and every study participant or their legally acceptable representative. The exact modalities and documentation of the informed consent should conform to local and national guidelines.

In India, all clinical research must conform to the National Ethical Guidelines for Biomedical and Health Research Involving Human Participants published by the Indian Council of Medical Research (ICMR), the last major revision of which was in 2017, as well as the New Drugs and Clinical Trial Rules (NDCT 2019) that was Gazette notified in 2019. There are separate versions of the guidelines for research involving children and research related to stem cells, and regenerative medicine. In all published work, the guidelines followed must be explicitly stated.

Current guidelines also make it mandatory that all clinical trials conducted in India must be registered prospectively with the Clinical Trial Registry of India (CTRI). Journals generally require, in consonance with ICMJE guidelines, that the registration number be communicated in the paper.

ACCESS TO RAW DATA

Access to raw data generated through research work not only allows journals to independently verify the accuracy of analysis but can also be of service to the broader scientific community if such data are shared with other researchers. Many reputed journals now require a data sharing statement from authors specifying whether individual deidentified participant data (including data dictionaries) will be shared and in what format, whether additional related documents will be available (e.g., study protocol and statistical analysis plan), when the data will become available and for how long, and by what access criteria data will be shared (including with whom, for what types of analyses, and by what mechanism). Public repositories of data can, in turn, spawn meaningful secondary research.

REPORTING GUIDELINES

Reporting guidelines have been developed for different study designs, and the largest repository of such guidelines, the online Enhancing the QUAlity and Transparency Of health Research (EQUATOR) Network (www.equator-network.org) provides access to 600 major and minor guidelines. The commonly used guidelines are listed in **Table 1**. Journals encourage authors to follow these reporting guidelines as they enhance reporting quality and ensure enough details for the work to be duly evaluated by editors, reviewers, and other researchers going through the published papers. Authors of review articles are encouraged to describe the methods used for locating, selecting, extracting, and synthesizing data.

TABLE 1: Popular reporting guidelines for biomedical research.

Research	Reporting guidelines
Randomized trials	CONSORT
Observational studies	STROBE
Systematic reviews and meta-analyses	PRISMA
Study protocols	SPIRIT, PRISMA-p
Diagnostic/Prognostic studies	STARD, TRIPOD
Case reports	CARE
Clinical practice guidelines	AGREE, RIGHT
Qualitative research	SRQR, COREQ
Quality improvement studies	SQUIRE
Economic evaluations	CHEERS
Animal/Preclinical studies	ARRIVE

As an illustrative example, let us consider the CONSORT (consolidated standards of reporting trials) statement. Randomized controlled trials represent the gold standard of clinical experimentation, and the CONSORT were developed to standardize and improve the quality of reporting of such experiments. The current CONSORT checklist includes 25 items (some with subitems) that address the methodology of clinical trial conduct so that no vital information is missed while reporting, and the whole serves as a ready reckoner for all stakeholders. The 2010 CONSORT checklist is reproduced in **Table 2.**

The CONSORT participant flow diagram template is provided in **Flowchart 1**.

ABBREVIATIONS AND SYMBOLS

Abbreviations can save space and word counts. It is generally recommended that authors use only standard abbreviations and avoid confusing the reader with nonstandard abbreviations. Also, most abbreviations are to be avoided in the title of the manuscript. Less common abbreviations to be used in the text should be spelled out in full at the first occurrence.

Guidelines regarding some other types of abbreviations are as follows:

- *Measurement units:* Journals may recommend the use of SI units. If these are not used exclusively, authors may provide the SI value in parentheses.
- *Drug names:* Provide the Recommended International Nonproprietary Name (rINN) in general. Additionally, brand names may be added if they are essential to interpretation of the results.

TABLE 2: CONSORT 2010 checklist.[4]

Section/Topic	Item No.	Checklist item	Reported on page
Title and abstract			
	1a	Identification as a randomized trial in the title	
	1b	Structured summary of trial design, methods, results, and conclusions (for specific guidance, see CONSORT for abstracts)	
Introduction			
Background and objectives	2a	Scientific background and explanation of the rationale	
	2b	Specific objectives or hypotheses	
Methods			
Trial design	3a	Description of trial design (such as parallel and factorial) including allocation ratio	
	3b	Important changes to methods after trial commencement (such as eligibility criteria), with reasons	
Participants	4a	Eligibility criteria for participants	
	4b	Settings and locations where the data were collected	
Interventions	5	The interventions for each group with sufficient details to allow replication, including how and when they were actually administered	
Outcomes	6a	Completely defined prespecified primary and secondary outcome measures, including how and when they were assessed	
	6b	Any changes to trial outcomes after the trial commenced, with reasons	
Sample size	7a	How sample size was determined	
	7b	When applicable, explanation of any interim analyses and stopping guidelines	
Randomization			
Sequence generation	8a	The method used to generate the random allocation sequence	
	8b	Type of randomization and details of any restriction (such as blocking and block size)	
Allocation concealment mechanism	9	The mechanism used to implement the random allocation sequence (such as sequentially numbered containers) and describing any steps taken to conceal the sequence until interventions were assigned	

Continued

Continued

Section/Topic	Item No.	Checklist item	Reported on page
Implementation	10	Who generated the random allocation sequence, who enrolled participants, and who assigned participants to interventions?	
Blinding	11a	If done, who was blinded after assignment to interventions (e.g., participants, care providers, and those assessing outcomes) and how?	
	11b	If relevant, a description of the similarity of interventions	
Statistical methods	12a	Statistical methods used to compare groups for primary and secondary outcomes	
	12b	Methods for additional analyses, such as subgroup analyses and adjusted analyses	
Results			
Participant flow (diagram strongly recommended)	13a	For each group, the number of participants who were randomly assigned, received intended treatment, and were analyzed for the primary outcome?	
	13b	For each group, losses and exclusions after randomization, together with reasons	
Recruitment	14a	Dates defining the periods of recruitment and follow-up	
	14b	Why the trial ended or was stopped?	
Baseline data	15	A table showing baseline demographic and clinical characteristics for each group	
Numbers analyzed	16	For each group, the number of participants (denominator) included in each analysis and whether the analysis was by originally assigned groups	
Outcomes and estimation	17a	For each primary and secondary outcome, results for each group, and the estimated effect size and its precision (such as 95% confidence interval)	
	17b	For binary outcomes, presentation of both absolute and relative effect sizes is recommended	
Ancillary analyses	18	Results of any other analyses performed, including subgroup analyses and adjusted analyses, distinguishing prespecified from exploratory	
Harms	19	All important harms or unintended effects in each group (for specific guidance, see CONSORT for harms)	

Continued

Continued

Section/Topic	Item No.	Checklist item	Reported on page
Discussion			
Limitations	20	Trial limitations, addressing sources of potential bias, imprecision, and, if relevant, multiplicity of analyses	
Generalizability	21	Generalizability (external validity and applicability) of the trial findings	
Interpretation	22	Interpretation consistent with results, balancing benefits and harms, and considering other relevant evidence	
Other information			
Registration	23	Registration number and name of trial registry	
Protocol	24	Where the full trial protocol can be accessed, if available	
Funding	25	Sources of funding and other support (such as supply of drugs) and role of funders	

(CONSORT: consolidated standards of reporting trials)
Source: Schulz et al. (2010).

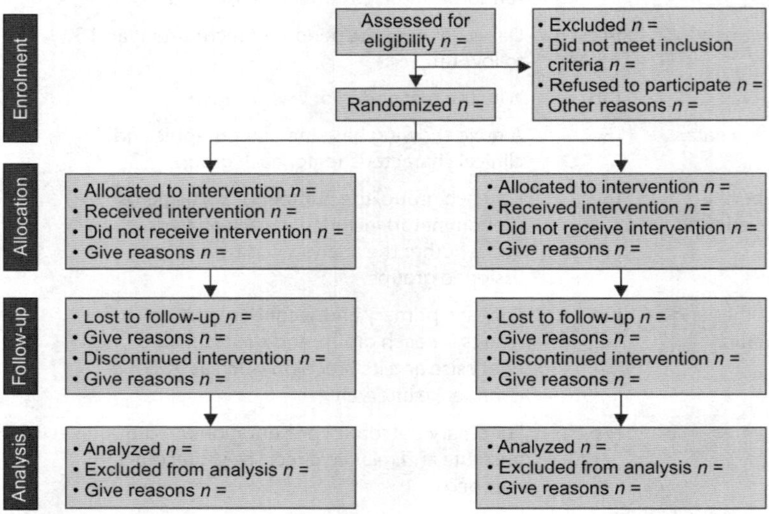

FLOWCHART 1: The CONSORT participant flow diagram.
(CONSORT: consolidated standards of reporting trials)

- *Species names:* These are written in italics (e.g., *Escherichia coli*). Write out in full the genus and species, both in the title of the manuscript and at the first mention of an organism in a paper. After the first mention, the genus name may be shortened to the first letter keeping the species name intact (e.g., *E. coli*).

- *Genes, mutations, genotypes, and alleles:* These are written in italics. Use the recommended name by consulting the appropriate genetic nomenclature database [e.g., HUGO Gene Nomenclature Committee (HGNC) for human genes]. It is sometimes advisable to indicate the synonyms for the gene the first time it appears in the text. Gene prefixes such as those used for oncogenes or cellular localization should be shown in roman typeface (e.g., *v-fes*, *c-MYC).*

FIGURES AND ILLUSTRATIONS[5]

Figures and illustrations in the form of graphs (plots), diagrams, or images (photographs) not only improve the presentation quality of scientific reporting but also enable a clear idea of many issues, particularly results, while reducing the length of the main text. To this end journals encourage the use of figures, but with limitations in respect of number that can be accommodated commensurate with article type. Individual journals have their own requirements regarding presentations of figures, but the following generally apply:

- All artworks must be the original work of the authors. In case figures published earlier are being reproduced in full or part, it is the authors' responsibility to secure the necessary permission from the copyright holder, unless they are open access.
- Figures are now submitted in digital format. Simple graphs, flowcharts, and diagrams may be incorporated in text documents such as those in MS-Word doc or Adobe pdf format, but more complex illustrations and photographic images are to be submitted in dedicated graphics formats such as bmp, jpg/jpeg, png, tiff, or cdx formats. The last is the ChemDraw format suitable for molecular structures.
- Authors should aim for the maximum image quality (resolution) within the constraint of maximum file size imposed by the journal. Generally, <600 dpi is not acceptable for photographic images.
- Figures are to be numbered in the order in which they are first mentioned in the text and uploaded in this order. Multipanel figures (those with parts a, b, c, etc.) need to be submitted as a single composite image that contains all parts of the figure.
- Figures should be uploaded in the correct orientation. Figure titles and legends are provided in the main manuscript, not in the graphic file. However, figure keys like letters, numbers, arrows or other pointers, symbols, scale bars, etc., are to be incorporated in the graphic itself.
- Although some journals redraw figures, many do not. However, journals usually will reduce figure size to match their column or page dimensions. Authors should crop their images to focus on the area of interest and make sure that symbols and annotations placed in the figure itself are clearly visible at these reduced dimensions.

- Some journals will require the submission of high-quality photoprints for things like radiographic scans, photomicrographs, blots, and other diagnostic imagery. Remember that illustrations submitted in color may lose contrast if not printed in color. Authors should consult journals regarding their color reproduction policy. Colored images in print journals may call for enhanced article processing charges.

Finally, it is also the responsibility of the author to ensure that appropriate photographic consent has been obtained if images with potentially identifiable features are to be published.

REFERENCING[6-8]

Referencing is a standardized way of acknowledging the sources of ideas and information used in planning, conducting, and interpreting research work. Adequate and accurate referencing is the responsibility of the authors, and it not only enhances the value of their presentation but also enables readers to understand the work and delve deeper into the subject. On the other hand, inadequate referencing may lead to accusations of plagiarism.

Journals vary in their policy regarding what can be cited and the format for citations, but the following are generally applicable:

- Unpublished papers, abstracts, data, and personal communications are generally not to be included in the reference list. Some journals may allow "unpublished observations" or "personal communication" to be cited in the main text, giving the names of the involved researchers. Obtaining permission to quote unpublished data or personal communications from colleagues is the responsibility of the author.
- There are different "styles" of citing published work but the Vancouver style of referencing recommended by ICMJE is now commonly followed. This is a numerical citation style where references in text, tables, and figures are numbered, consecutively in the order they appear, using numbers in parentheses or superscript and then listed in that order in the references section.
- Formats are standardized for citing many different sources of information, including journal articles, books, book chapters, monographs, conference abstracts, theses, newspaper articles, electronic storage media, webpages, data repositories, and various other internet sources. The United States National Library of Medicine (US-NLM) has published a detailed guide in this regard that is periodically updated.
- Journal names are abbreviated in citations to a standard format as recommended by US-NLM in their cataloging service. Publication locations are included if journals of the same name are published in more than one city.
- Other common referencing styles for biomedical literature are the Harvard style and the American Psychological Association (APA) style.

All web links and URLs should be given a reference number and included in the reference list rather than within the text of the manuscript. While referencing they should be cited in appropriate style along with the date on which they were last accessed. The latter is important as web link contents may disappear or undergo major modification without notice. The authors should, therefore, archive a dated copy of the web pages they are using as references.

The use of reference manager software can simplify the task of collating and formatting citations. These software allow one to collect references, store references and notes, organize references, format references in a required referencing style to create a reference list or bibliography, and insert in-text citations into a document as it is being generated. BibBase, Bookends, EndNote, RefWorks, Mendeley, Zotero, etc., are examples of such software. Some like BibBase, Mendeley, and Zotero are free, while others like Bookends, EndNote, and RefWorks are paid or subscription based.

CONCLUSION

Despite the availability of publication guidelines for many years, the quality of reporting of research studies, particularly those published from India, is often not up to the mark. Awareness of these reporting guidelines has been suboptimal. Coupled with enhanced efforts on the part of the journal community to improve awareness, what is needed is self-education of the research community is needed regarding the importance and modalities of achieving better reporting quality.

- Publication guidelines facilitate the writing of scientific reports and enhance the quality of reporting. The Recommendations for the Conduct, Reporting, Editing, and Publication of Scholarly Work in Medical Journals framed by the ICMJE are now widely followed. They were last updated in January 2024.
- The guidelines cover a range of issues related to the roles and responsibilities of various stakeholders, process of framing, submitting, peer review, publication of the report, and many allied aspects such as ethical safeguards for research participants, clinical trial registration, publication ethics, sponsorships, and copyright issues.
- ICMJE has clearly defined authorship criteria that are now almost universally accepted.
- Now, many reporting guidelines exist to facilitate quality reporting of different types of clinical and preclinical research. One of the most widely used such guidelines is the CONSORT statement for reporting clinical trials.
- Authors need to be conversant with the correct use of abbreviations, tables, and figures in their manuscripts. Figure quality has to be given a lot of attention for precise and legible reproduction in the published paper.

- Of the different referencing styles available, the Vancouver style has become the most widely used. The use of reference manager software can simplify the task of collating and formatting citations.
- The quality of scientific reporting is still suboptimal in many cases and quality improvement will require greater awareness of publication guidelines and greater self-learning of the research community.

REFERENCES

1. International Committee of Medical Journal Editors. (2024). Recommendations for the conduct, reporting, editing, and publication of scholarly work in medical journals. [online] Available from https://www.icmje.org/recommendations/ [Last accessed February, 2024].
2. Ali MJ. ICMJE criteria for authorship: Why the criticisms are not justified? Graefes Arch Clin Exp Ophthalmol. 2021;259:289-90.
3. Matheson, A. The ICMJE Recommendations and pharmaceutical marketing–strengths, weaknesses and the unsolved problem of attribution in publication ethics. BMC Med Ethics. 2016;17:20.
4. Schulz KF, Altman DG, Moher D; CONSORT Group. CONSORT 2010 Statement: Updated guidelines for reporting parallel group randomised trials. BMC Med. 2010;8:18.
5. Wang SC. Preparing effective medical illustrations for publication (Part 1): Pixel-based image acquisition. Biomed Imaging Interv J. 2008;4(1):e11.
6. Patrias K. In: Wendling DL (Ed). Citing Medicine: The NLM Style Guide for Authors, Editors, And Publishers, 2nd edition. Bethesda, MD: National Library of Medicine (US); 2007. [online] Available from http://www.nlm.nih.gov/citingmedicine [Last accessed February, 2024].
7. Wikipedia, The Free Encyclopedia. (2024). Comparison of reference management software. [online] Available from https://en.wikipedia.org/wiki/Comparison_of_reference_management_software [Last accessed February, 2024].
8. Menon V. Beyond research reporting guidelines: How can the quality of published research be enhanced? Indian J Psychol Med. 2019;41:303-5.

3

SECTION

Manuscript Submission

CHAPTER 11

An Overview of Manuscript Preparation

Mangesh Tiwaskar, Agam Vora, Rakesh Bhadade

INTRODUCTION

Publication in the medical field is a cornerstone of scientific progress and dissemination of knowledge. In this chapter, we will try to explore the nuances and intricacies of the *art of publication* in the medical field. From the need for publication to the various aspects of writing, selecting the right journal or publication platform, addressing issues of copyrights, plagiarism, concealing personal details, and proper referencing, we will try to delve into the fundamental principles and best practices in medical publishing.

In the 21st century, the field of medicine is marked by rapid developments in diagnosis, treatment, and overall patient care. Researchers, clinicians, and healthcare professionals are constantly in a quest to enhance medical knowledge, with the goal of improving patient outcomes and the quality of healthcare. The dissemination of medical knowledge is an essential part of this process.

EVOLVING LANDSCAPE OF MEDICAL PUBLICATION

The landscape of medical publication has evolved significantly over the years, influenced by technological advancements and changes in the healthcare industry. Traditional print journals are no longer the sole means of disseminating medical research. Digital platforms, open-access journals, and preprint servers have emerged as powerful tools for sharing knowledge. This shift has both benefits and challenges, which we will discuss in subsequent sections.[1]

Need for Publication[1]

Why should medical professionals and researchers embark on the journey of publication in the first place? Understanding the compelling reasons for publishing in the medical field is the foundation of successful medical research dissemination.

- *Contribution to medical knowledge*: Publication is a primary means of contributing to the vast reservoir of medical knowledge. Research findings, clinical insights, and innovations are useless if they remain confined to the source of origin. Through publication, you have the opportunity to share your discoveries with the medical community, potentially benefiting patients worldwide.
- *Scientific and clinical progress*: The medical field is dynamic and ever-evolving. New diseases emerge, treatment approaches change, and diagnostic methods improve. By publishing your research and experiences, you actively participate in advancing scientific and clinical progress. Your work may lead to new treatments, diagnostic tools, or medical guidelines that improve patient outcomes.
- *Peer recognition and collaboration*: Publishing your research allows your peers to recognize your expertise and contributions. It can open doors to collaboration with other researchers and institutions. Collaboration often leads to more significant discoveries and a broader impact on the medical field.
- *Personal and professional growth*: A robust publication record can significantly enhance your career in the medical field. Whether you are a medical student, resident, clinician, or researcher, publishing is a mark of achievement and expertise. It can lead to promotions, tenure, and opportunities to lead medical research projects.
- *Addressing clinical challenges*: Medical professionals face daily challenges in patient care. By publishing your clinical experiences, you can help address common clinical challenges. Your insights may inspire innovative solutions that benefit not only your practice but also the broader medical community.
- *Ethical responsibility*: In healthcare, ethical responsibility extends beyond patient care. It includes sharing knowledge that can save lives, improve health outcomes, and prevent suffering. Publishing in the medical field aligns with this ethical duty to contribute to the greater good.
- *Bridging gaps in healthcare*: Medical publication can bridge the gaps in healthcare by disseminating best practices, guidelines, and research to underserved regions and populations. It contributes to reducing healthcare disparities and improving global health equity.

ART OF WRITING THE MANUSCRIPT[2,3]

The art of writing a medical manuscript is a multifaceted process that involves not only conveying your research findings but also adhering to established conventions and ethical standards. In this section, we will explore the key components of crafting a compelling and impactful medical publication.

- *Define your objectives*: Before you begin writing your manuscript, it is crucial to clarify your objectives. What do you hope to achieve with this publication? Is it to present original research, share clinical experiences, or review existing literature? Defining your objectives will guide the structure and content of your manuscript.
- *Structure your manuscript*: A well-structured manuscript is easier to read and comprehend. Most medical manuscripts follow a standard structure:
    - Title: Your title should be concise, informative, and attention-grabbing.
    - Abstract: Summarize your research, methodology, key results, and implications in a structured abstract.
    - Introduction: Provide context, explain the problem or research question, and state the purpose of your study.
    - Methods: Describe your research design, data collection methods, and statistical analysis.
    - Results: Present your findings objectively and concisely. Use tables and figures to enhance clarity.
    - Discussion: Interpret your results, discuss their implications, and relate them to existing literature.
    - Conclusion: Summarize the main findings and their significance.
    - References: Cite all sources used in your manuscript following a recognized citation style [e.g., American Medical Association (AMA), American Psychological Association (APA), or Vancouver].
- *Write clearly and concisely*: Effective medical writing demands clarity and conciseness. Avoid jargon and overly technical language. Explain complex concepts in simple terms to ensure that your manuscript is accessible to a broad audience, including clinicians, researchers, and students.
- *Use evidence-based language*: Medical writing relies on evidence-based language. Support your statements with appropriate citations from reputable sources. Be cautious with making claims that are not substantiated by solid evidence.
- *Ethical considerations*: Medical writing comes with ethical responsibilities. Disclose conflicts of interest, funding sources, and ethical approval for research involving human or animal subjects. Maintain patient confidentiality and adhere to guidelines like the Declaration of Helsinki.
- *Collaborate and seek feedback*: Collaboration can enhance the quality of your manuscript. Collaborate with colleagues and mentors for critical feedback. Peer review helps identify weaknesses and ensures the scientific rigor of your work.
- *Address the peer-review process*: Anticipate peer review, which is a crucial step in the publication process. Address reviewers' comments professionally and thoroughly. A successful peer review will lead to publication in reputable journals.

METHOD OF JOURNAL SELECTION OR PUBLICATION PLATFORM SELECTION[4]

Selecting the right journal or publication platform is a vital decision that impacts the reach and visibility of your work. Here is how to navigate this process effectively:

- *Define your target audience*: Identify your target audience—clinicians, researchers, educators, residents, students, or the public. Consider which audience will benefit most from your research or insights.
- *Impact factor and reputation*: Consider the impact factor and reputation of the journal. The impact factor is a measure of a journal's influence in the field. Reputable journals with high impact factors are often preferred for original research. But be informed that submission of your research to low impact factor journals may minimize the chances of rejection.
- *Open-access journals*: Open-access journals provide unrestricted access to your work, ensuring a broader readership. However, be aware of publication fees associated with some open-access journals.
- *Specialty versus general journals*: Choose between specialty and general medical journals. Specialty journals may be ideal for research specific to a particular medical field, while general journals offer broader exposure.
- *Review author guidelines*: Review the author guidelines provided by the journal or publication platform. Ensure that your manuscript complies with their formatting and submission requirements.
- *Peer-review process*: Understand the journal's peer-review process. Rigorous peer review is a hallmark of reputable journals, ensuring the quality and credibility of published work.
- *Copyright and licensing*: Determine the journal's policies on copyright and licensing. You should retain the right to share your work and findings freely, particularly in the case of open-access journals.
- *Consider alternative platforms*: Explore alternative publication platforms, such as preprint servers, which provide immediate access to your work. These platforms are increasingly popular for rapid dissemination of research.

Selecting the right journal or publication platform is a crucial step in the publication process. It directly influences the visibility and impact of your research or clinical insights. Take the time to make an informed decision and consider seeking guidance from mentors or colleagues with publishing experience.

COPYRIGHTS

Copyrights protect the intellectual property of authors. In medical publication, the following points should be taken care of.

- *Ownership of copyright*: Authors typically retain the copyright to their work. However, some journals or publishers may require authors to

transfer copyright. Ensure that you understand and agree with the terms of the publication agreement.
- *Licensing*: Choose a suitable license for your work. Open-access journals often require a creative commons license, which permits broad sharing and reuse. Different licenses have varying conditions, so make an informed choice.
- *Republishing rights*: Review the journal's policies on republishing your work. Some journals may restrict or impose conditions on republishing. It is essential to know if you can share your research elsewhere, like on your personal website or in institutional repositories.
- *Ethical and legal considerations*: Always adhere to ethical and legal guidelines regarding copyright. Avoid using copyrighted images or content without proper permission or attribution. Cite sources diligently, ensuring that your manuscript complies with copyright laws. Images, figures, tables, or literature freely available on internet may not necessarily be free to reuse or republish.

PLAGIARISM[5]

Plagiarism is a serious ethical breach that can have severe consequences in medical publishing. Preventing plagiarism involves the following practices.
- *Cite sources properly*: Accurately and consistently cite all sources, including text, figures, and tables. Adhere to a recognized citation style, such as AMA, APA, or Vancouver, and follow the specific journal's guidelines for citation and referencing.
- *Use plagiarism detection software*: Prior to submission, employ plagiarism detection tools to check your manuscript. These tools can identify any instances of unoriginal content and help you correct or attribute them appropriately.
- *Paraphrase and attribute*: When using someone else's work, paraphrase and attribute it accurately. Clearly reference the original source, even when paraphrasing, to give proper credit.
- *Self-plagiarism*: Be aware of self-plagiarism, where you reuse your own previous work without proper citation. Different journals have varying policies on self-plagiarism, so it is essential to understand and follow these guidelines.

PATIENT PRIVACY AND CONFIDENTIALITY[6]

Protecting patient privacy and confidentiality is an ethical obligation in medical publishing. To ensure patient confidentiality:
- *De-identify patient information*: Remove or de-identify any personal or identifying information about patients in your manuscript. This includes names, dates of birth, and other demographic details that could reveal their identity.

- *Informed consent*: If your manuscript includes case details or information about patients, ensure that you have obtained informed consent from the individuals involved. Properly document the consent process to demonstrate ethical compliance.
- *Institutional Review Board (IRB) approval*: For research involving human subjects, it is crucial to obtain IRB approval. Mention this approval in your manuscript to indicate that your research adheres to ethical oversight and legal regulations.

REFERENCING

Accurate and comprehensive referencing is fundamental to maintaining the integrity of your medical publication:

- *Citation style*: Adhere to the designated citation style for the journal you are submitting to. This consistency in citation style enhances the clarity and professionalism of your manuscript.
- *Organize references*: Create a reference list organized alphabetically. Ensure that each citation within your text corresponds to a complete and correctly formatted reference in the list.
- *Verify accuracy*: Thoroughly check each reference for accuracy. Ensure that page numbers, DOIs (Digital Object Identifiers), and other relevant details are correct. Inaccurate referencing can impact the credibility of your work.
- *Use citation management tools*: Citation management tools like EndNote or Mendeley can be valuable in simplifying the citation process. These tools help format references and generate bibliographies efficiently.

CONCLUSION

The conclusion of your medical manuscript is your final opportunity to leave a lasting impact on your readers:

- *Summarize key findings*: Provide a concise summary of the primary findings of your study or clinical report. Emphasize the significance and practical implications of these findings.
- *Address limitations*: Acknowledge any limitations of your research or study. Transparency about limitations is a mark of scientific integrity and helps readers interpret your results appropriately.
- *Future directions*: Discuss potential future research or clinical implications of your work. Suggest avenues for further exploration in the field, which can inspire other researchers and clinicians.
- *Reflect on the impact*: Conclude by reflecting on the broader impact of your research or clinical insights. Explain how your work contributes to the field of medicine and patient care. Convey the importance of your findings in advancing medical knowledge.

KEY TAKEAWAYS[7]

Need for Publication

- Medical publication is essential for advancing medical knowledge, peer review, clinical guidance, education, and professional growth.
- It is an ethical responsibility in healthcare to share knowledge and contribute to the greater good.
- Medical publication can help bridge healthcare gaps and reduce disparities.

Art of Writing the Manuscript

- Define your objectives before starting to write.
- Follow a structured format for your manuscript, including a title, abstract, introduction, methods, results, discussion, conclusion, and references.
- Write clearly and concisely, avoiding jargon and technical language.
- Use evidence-based language and support your claims with citations.
- Collaborate and seek feedback from peers and mentors.
- Anticipate the peer-review process and address reviewers' comments professionally.

Method of Journal Selection or Publication Platform Selection

- Define your target audience to select the right journal or platform.
- Consider factors like impact factor, reputation, open-access availability, and focus (specialty vs. general).
- Review the journal's author guidelines, peer-review process, and copyright and licensing policies.
- Ensure you have the right to republish or share your work.
- Explore alternative platforms like preprint servers for rapid dissemination.

Copyrights

- Understand the ownership and licensing of copyrights for your publication.
- Choose the right license for your work, considering the terms and conditions.
- Be aware of republishing rights and restrictions.
- Adhere to ethical and legal guidelines regarding copyright, avoiding the use of copyrighted material without proper permission or attribution.

Plagiarism

- Cite sources properly and consistently using a recognized citation style.
- Use plagiarism detection software to check your manuscript for unoriginal content.

- Paraphrase and attribute content from other sources correctly.
- Be cautious of self-plagiarism, which can be subject to journal-specific policies.

Concealing Personal Details

- De-identify patient information to protect privacy and confidentiality.
- Obtain informed consent when including case details or patient information.
- Ensure that research involving human subjects has received IRB approval.

Referencing

- Use the designated citation style specified by the journal.
- Organize references alphabetically and ensure that all citations correspond to complete and accurately formatted references.
- Verify the accuracy of each reference, including page numbers and DOIs.
- Consider using citation management tools to streamline the process.

Conclusion[8]

- Summarize key findings in the conclusion.
- Address limitations transparently.
- Suggest future directions for research or clinical practice.
- Reflect on the broader impact of your work on the field of medicine and patient care.

By following these key takeaways and best practices, you can effectively contribute to the advancement of medical knowledge and the betterment of healthcare through your publications.

REFERENCES

1. http://www.mciindia.org/RulesandRegulations/TeachersEligibilityQualifications1998.aspx.
2. Fishbein M (Ed). An acceptable paper. In: Medical Writing, 3rd edition. York: The Maple Press Company; 1957. pp. 1-4.
3. Fishbein M (Ed). Construction of the manuscript. In: Medical Writing, 3rd edition. York: The Maple Press Company; 1957. pp. 34-40.
4. Elsaie ML, Kammer J. Impactitis: The impact factor myth syndrome. Indian J Dermatol. 2009;54:83-5.
5. Singh A, Singh M, Singh AK, Singh D, Singh P, Sharma A. Free full text articles: Where to search for them? Int J Trichol. 2011;3:75-9.
6. Klinger JK, Scanlon D, Pressley M. How to publish in scholarly journals. Educ Res. 2005;34(8):14-20.
7. Jones R. Choosing a research question. Asia Pac Fam Med. 2003;2:42-4.
8. Madke B, Khopkar U. Get set, write. Indian J Dermatol Venereol Leprol. 2011;77:392-8.

CHAPTER 12

How to Choose a Journal?

Jyotirmoy Pal, Nandini Chatterjee, Mangesh Tiwaskar

INTRODUCTION

Journals have served as the mouthpiece of research work for more than three and a half centuries. But in today's technological world, there is an explosion of journals and it is difficult to identify the right journal to publish research.

The landscape of medical publication has evolved significantly over the years, influenced by technological advancements and changes in the healthcare industry. Traditional print journals are no longer the sole means of disseminating medical research. Digital platforms, open-access journals, and preprint servers have emerged as powerful tools for sharing knowledge. This shift has both benefits and challenges, which we will discuss in subsequent sections.

Selecting the right journal or publication platform is a vital decision that impacts the reach and visibility of your work.

There are certain issues to be resolved which are mentioned as follows:[1]

- It is important to find a journal with a wide reach, low chance of rejection, and less time for publication.
- It is also considered whether the journal reach the target audience.
- The journal has to be legitimate and likely to help in the advancement of ones' career.

The criteria for evaluating a journal are the following:[2]

- Academic credibility
- Peer review process
- Publication ethics
- Editorial board members
- Journal reputation
- Copyright issues
- Indexing status
- Impact factor
- Operational issues

HOW TO NAVIGATE THE PROCESS OF JOURNAL SELECTION EFFECTIVELY?[3]

Define Your Target Audience

Identify your target audience—clinicians, researchers, educators, residents, students, or the public. Consider which audience will benefit most from your research or insights.

Impact Factor and Reputation[4]

Consider the impact factor and reputation of the journal. The impact factor is a measure of a journal's influence in the field. Reputable journals with high impact factors are often preferred for original research. But be informed, submission of your research to low-impact-factor journals may minimize the chances of rejection. One should also review the *editorial board members* that can reveal valuable insights of journal. Credential of editor in chief and contact information of editorial staffs and office address should be noted for assessing credibility of a journal.

Open-access Journals

Open-access journals provide unrestricted access to your work, ensuring a broader readership. However, be aware of publication fees associated with some open-access journals.

Specialty versus General Journals

Choose between specialty and general medical journals. Specialty journals may be ideal for research specific to a particular medical field, while general journals offer broader exposure. Exemplary research may also be rejected if the issue does not fall within the scope of the journal.

Every journal's homepage has a section named "About the Journal". This helps to have a clear idea of the aims and scope of a journal. In addition previous published articles are to be reviewed for this purpose.

Review Author Guidelines

Review the author guidelines provided by the journal or publication platform. Ensure your manuscript complies with their formatting and submission requirements.

Peer Review Process

Understand the journal's peer review process. Rigorous peer review is a hallmark of reputable journals, ensuring the quality and credibility of published work.

Indexing Status

This is important for articles to be discoverable and read by others. Proper indexing of journals adds to their reputation in terms of broad coverage in reputed databases.

The databases consider the peer review process, regularity of publication, and reputation of journal or mother body before indexing the journal.

MEDLINE, SCOPUS, EMBASE, DOAJ, etc., are important indexing agencies which are recognized by the National Medical Commission (NMC).

Copyright and Licensing

Determine the journal's policies on copyright and licensing. You should retain the right to share your work and findings freely, particularly in the case of open-access journals.

Publishing Time and Acceptance Rate

These need to be assessed before submission depending upon your urgency for publication.

Consider Alternative Platforms

Explore alternative publication platforms, such as preprint servers, which provide immediate access to your work. These platforms are increasingly popular for rapid dissemination of research.

To be Wary of Predatory Journals[5,6]

Some of the clues to predatory journals are:

- Quick publication
- Vague policies of plagiarism check, retraction, and corrections
- Absence of proper peer review
- Manuscripts are received via email rather than the online submission tool.
- Unclear copyright policy
- Article processing and/or publication fee is nominal.
- There is no information available regarding the preservation and archiving of journal content.
- The journal's scope is not clearly delineated.
- There are grammatical and typographical errors on the website.

CONCLUSION

Selecting the right journal or publication platform is a crucial step in the publication process. It directly influences the visibility and impact of your research or clinical insights. Take the time to make an informed decision, and consider seeking guidance from mentors or colleagues with publishing experience.

REFERENCES

1. Committee of Medical Journal Editors (ICMJE). (2024). Recommendations for the Conduct, Reporting, Editing, and Publication of Scholarly Work in Medical Journals. [online] Available from http://www.icmje.org/icmje-recommendations.pdf [Last accessed January, 2024].
2. Suiter AM, Sarli CC. Selecting a Journal for Publication: Criteria to Consider. Mo Med. 2019;116(6):461-5.
3. EQUATOR Network. Enhancing the Quality and Transparency of Health Research (Equator) Reporting Guidelines. [online] Available from https://www.equator-network.org/reporting-guidelines/ [Last accessed January, 2024].
4. Garfield E. The Agony and the Ecstasy—The History and Meaning of the Journal Impact Factor. Paper presented at: Chicago: International Congress on Peer Review and Biomedical Publication; 2005.
5. Beall J. Predatory publishers are corrupting open access. Nature. Nature. 2012;489:179.
6. Cobey KD, Lalu MM, Skidmore B, Ahmadzai N, Grudniewicz A, Moher D. What is a predatory journal? A scoping review. F1000Res. 2018;7:1001.

CHAPTER 13

Journal Metrics Made Easy

Shambo Samrat Samajdar, Santanu K Tripathi, Shreyashi Dasgupta

INTRODUCTION

For healthcare professionals, the landscape of academic literature can appear vast and intricate. Deciphering the merit and relevance of various scientific journals becomes critical, particularly when considering where to publish or which research to cite. In an evolving digital landscape, the methods used to measure the influence and relevance of scientific research have also transformed. Gone are the days when the solitary benchmark for gauging the success or influence of a journal article rested solely on traditional metrics. While these metrics, especially the widely recognized journal impact factor (JIF), have long held sway in the academic world, they are not without their limitations, often giving a narrowed view of an article's overall impact and sometimes misleading research evaluations and academic promotions.[1]

The digital age, characterized by the rapid proliferation of online resources and a more interconnected global community, has necessitated the advent of article-level metrics (ALM). These metrics are gaining traction as more holistic and immediate indicators of the dissemination and impact of scientific information. Traditional metrics, like citations, often lag in reflecting the real-time significance and scholarly application of articles. In contrast, several new-age metrics, often termed "alternative metrics" or "altmetrics", quickly pinpoint articles that resonate with audiences, thus enabling researchers and publishers to refine their strategies.[2]

Yet, it is crucial to recognize that all metrics, whether traditional or alternative, are intricately tied to how a journal is promoted and digitized, which in turn defines its readership and influence. The power of digitization is most evident when we consider the role of platforms like Altmetric.com and Plum Analytics. These platforms thrive on the assignment of digital object identifiers (DOIs) to articles, a simple yet transformative technology that greatly enhances the visibility and traceability of scientific research.[3] Astonishingly, a considerable fraction of articles, even in this digital age, remain without a DOI, with disparities observed across various countries. Interestingly, a review of 496,665 articles indexed in PubMed revealed that over the past half-century, a significant proportion (40.5%) of these articles were not assigned a DOI. This research further highlighted that the practice of DOI allocation was more prevalent in countries like the US, the UK, and the Netherlands compared to Russia, the Czech Republic, and Romania.[3]

Furthermore, the global shift toward digitization has reshaped how scholars select, categorize, and utilize scientific articles. With the integration of advanced digital tools in global databases like Scopus and PubMed, it is now feasible to track not just citations but the broader attention an article garners. This comprehensive approach provides scholars with insights into trending topics and influential articles in their respective fields.

Notably, experts in the realm of scientific publishing are welcoming the move toward ALM.[4] Platforms such as Mendeley, with its bookmarking counts, offer a promising alternative to traditional citation counts. These counts often accumulate faster, giving early indicators of an article's influence, even though not all bookmarks translate to eventual citations.[5]

With a diverse array of both established and emerging metrics under discussion, our aim in this chapter is to provide a thorough overview of ALM. We seek to shed light on their implications, strengths, and potential areas of enhancement, with the hope of equipping researchers, authors, and publishers with the knowledge to navigate this complex landscape effectively and delve deep into the intricacies of journal metrics, demystifying them for the benefit of the modern scholar.

UNDERSTANDING IMPACT FACTOR

What is Impact Factor?

The impact factor (IF), developed by the Institute for Scientific Information (ISI), is a widely recognized journal metric. It calculates the average number of citations received by articles published in a journal over the previous 2 years. For instance, if a journal's IF for 2023 is 5, on average, each article published in 2021 and 2022 was cited five times in 2023.

Interpretation in medicine: In the medical field, journals with a higher IF are typically seen as more influential. However, IF should be contextualized.

Discipline-specific variances: IF varies across medical specialties. A high IF in one field might be considered average in another.

Reading between the numbers: Some high-IF journals may prefer reviews or clinically oriented research, influencing the type of studies you might choose to submit.

Understanding the Journal Impact Factor

The JIF has been a cornerstone in the realm of scientific publishing. Its origins trace back to Eugene Garfield's 1955 proposal[6] in the journal "Science". Initially introduced as a tool to aid librarians in collection management, it has since evolved to become a significant yardstick in Scientometrics.

Origins and Evolution

Eugene Garfield envisioned the JIF as a means to assist librarians in selecting essential titles for their collections during the 1960s. Alongside Sher, he introduced the notion of JIF, which aided in recognizing journals that, despite publishing a few articles, were highly influential. Garfield's ventures did not stop there. He founded the "Institute for Scientific Information" and initiated the "Science Citation Index" (SCI) in 1964. With time, this expanded to include the Social Science Citation Index (SSCI) and the Art and Humanities Citation Index (AHCI). The underpinnings of citation networking and the significance of linking citations were largely conceptualized during this period.[7-9]

JIF: How is it Calculated?

This is a straightforward metric. It gauges the citations a journal receives in a specific year for articles from the prior 2 years. It is expressed as:

JIF = (Number of citations in a year for content from the previous 2 years)/
(Total articles and reviews from those 2 years)

Critique and Counterarguments

While JIF is widely accepted, it is not free from criticism:[10]

- *Quality versus quantity*: Detractors argue that JIF does not encapsulate the actual quality of an article. It offers average values, which can be influenced by a few articles. Moreover, the 2-year citation window may overlook impactful articles that gain recognition over a more extended period.
- *Potential for manipulation*: Journals might artificially inflate their JIF by publishing a higher number of review articles or by practices like self-citation.
- *Does not represent individual merit*: JIF might reflect a journal's standing, but it does not necessarily translate to the quality of an individual article or a researcher's contribution. Eugene Garfield himself stated the importance of evaluating the actual impact of individual papers over using JIF as a proxy.
- *Changing landscape of publishing*: With the rise of open-access platforms and preprint repositories, traditional metrics like JIF face challenges in capturing the complete spectrum of a paper's influence.

- *Language and field bias*: Critics point out the potential bias toward English language journals and differences in citation practices across various fields.

While the JIF is an established metric, it is crucial to use it judiciously. It serves as a tool, not a definitive measure. The emphasis should always be on the quality and integrity of scientific research. Embracing transparency, promoting ethical practices, and focusing on the broader goals of advancing knowledge will ensure that the JIF and other metrics are used to enhance, not hinder, the scientific community's progress.

OTHER KEY JOURNAL-LEVEL METRICS

SCImago Journal Rank

SCImago Journal Rank (SJR), powered by Scopus database information, measures the scientific influence of scholarly journals. It accounts not only for the number of citations but also for the prestige of the citing journals. Unlike the IF, SJR includes a wider range of citations (not limited to the previous 2 years) and is normalized by subject field.

Spotlight on SJR: SCImago Journal & Country Rank is a renowned tool, offering insights into the prestige and citation impact of scientific journals, using data derived from the Scopus database.

Why is SJR Important?

- *Accessibility*: SJR is a free and publicly available resource. Unlike some resources, it does not require a subscription.
- *Comprehensive coverage*: SJR ranks a wider range of journals than Journal Citation Reports, encompassing all academic disciplines.
- *Citation normalization*: SJR considers the variance in citation behaviors across different fields. To achieve this, it normalizes its rankings, ensuring fair comparisons.
- *Transfer of prestige*: At the core of SJR is the notion that not all citations carry the same weight. Citations from esteemed journals are given more importance compared to those from lesser-known journals. This idea mirrors how search engines, like Google, rank web pages based on the quality of their links.

Understanding the SJR Calculation

SCImago Journal Rank is not just about the frequency of citations, it is about the prestige associated with those citations. To put it simply, for a given journal, its SJR for 2020 would be computed as:
Weighted citations in 2020 to articles from 2019, 2018, and 2017 divided by (total articles published in 2019, 2018, and 2017)

Here is a deeper dive into what makes SJR distinct:

- *Reputation matters*: SJR values the reputation of the citing journal. This approach ensures a fair assessment among journals from different fields and of varying renown.
- *Holistic view on citations*: SJR does not just count citations, it weighs them based on the journal's prestige, offering a nuanced view of a journal's influence.
- *Citation pattern adjustment*: Recognizing that different fields have distinct citation behaviors, SJR adjusts its metrics accordingly, ensuring that journals from diverse disciplines can be fairly compared.
- *Minimized bias*: By valuing the prestige of citations, SJR diminishes the potential for editorial manipulation through self-citations.
- *Wide-ranging journal coverage*: The SJR includes a broad spectrum of journals, ensuring inclusive coverage, even extending to social sciences.
- *Updated frequency*: It is also worth noting that Scopus refreshes SJR values biannually, ensuring the most current and relevant insights.

Crafted by Félix de Moya, the SJR is a beacon in the realm of journal metrics, offering a more sophisticated and comprehensive measure of journal impact and quality. It transcends traditional IFs by adding a layer of prestige to the citation value, making it a pivotal tool in academic research and journal evaluation.[11]

CiteScore

CiteScore, also derived from the Scopus database, measures the average citations received per document in a 3-year period. It includes all document types (research articles, reviews, conference papers, etc.), providing a broader overview of a journal's impact.

A Comprehensive Approach to CiteScore

CiteScore is an innovative metric developed by Scopus, a renowned citation indexing database by Elsevier. Offering a transparent, comprehensive, and updated measure of a journal's impact, CiteScore analyzes citations over a 3-year period, as opposed to the 2-year span typically used by the JIF.

Why Choose CiteScore?

- *Accessibility*: No need for a Scopus subscription to access CiteScore rankings.
- *Broad coverage*: Ranks a wider array of journals than most other metrics.
- *Disciplinary diversity*: All academic fields are represented.
- *Extended analysis period*: The 4-year analysis provides a more representative overview of citation behavior.
- *Transparency*: The calculation methodology is open and easy to understand.

CiteScore Calculation

For CiteScore 2023:

A: Total citations from 2023 for documents published in 2020, 2021, and 2022.

B: Total documents published during 2020, 2021, and 2022.

The formula is: CiteScore 2023 value = A ÷ B

Factor	Description
A	Citations in 2023 to documents from 2020 to 2022
B	Total documents indexed in Scopus published between 2020 and 2022
CiteScore value	A ÷ B

Benefits of CiteScore[12,13]

- *Broad scope*: Includes all document types in both its numerator and denominator, offering a holistic view of a journal's impact.
- *Comprehensive*: Measures average citations per document for a title over a 3-year window, capturing both fast and slow-evolving fields.
- *Transparent calculation*: No hidden details or secret algorithms. CiteScore values are based on clear and replicable calculations.
- *Real-time tracking with CiteScore tracker*: Provides an ongoing view of a journal's performance during the year, updating monthly.
- *Swift inclusion of new titles*: Titles indexed by Scopus can receive CiteScore metrics the following year, ensuring contemporary relevancy.

CiteScore versus other metrics: While CiteScore is akin to other journal metrics, it stands out due to its broad inclusion criteria, encompassing not just articles and reviews, but also other document types like letters, notes, and conference papers. This gives a more rounded representation of a journal's impact. Plus, CiteScore, being part of Scopus's basket of journal metrics, also complements other metrics like SNIP and SJR, offering a complete picture of a journal's influence.

In summary, CiteScore provides an accessible, comprehensive, and transparent approach to journal metrics, making it an invaluable tool for researchers, authors, and institutions. With its clear calculation and broad scope, CiteScore is set to reshape our understanding of journal impact in the academic world.

Source Normalized Impact per Paper

Source Normalized Impact per Paper, often abbreviated as SNIP, stands out as a key metric for assessing the citation impact of scholarly journals. Developed by Professor Henk F Moed at the Centre for Science and Technology Studies (CWTS) of the University of Leiden, this metric offers a comprehensive perspective on the relevance and significance of journals in their respective scientific fields.

Understanding SNIP

Unlike conventional citation metrics, SNIP provides a more holistic view of a journal's impact. It places citations in context by accounting for the citation patterns and practices of various academic disciplines. This is particularly beneficial when comparing journals from different scientific fields, as citation frequencies and behaviors can differ greatly between them.

Key Features of SNIP

- *Contextual citation impact*: SNIP emphasizes the importance of the context in which a citation occurs. Not all citations carry the same weight. In fields where citations are less common, each citation holds greater significance, and vice versa.
- *Research field's citation frequency*: By taking into account the typical citation frequency of a specific research domain, SNIP ensures that journals are evaluated on a level playing field.
- *Normalization*: SNIP does not solely rely on raw citation counts. Instead, it "normalizes" these figures based on the citation behavior of a field. This ensures fairness in assessment.
- *Independence from subject classification*: To sidestep potential biases, SNIP calculations do not lean on a journal's subject classification.
- *Transparency against editorial manipulation*: Designed to be robust, the SNIP metric minimizes the chances of editorial interference influencing the score.

SNIP's Evolution

Initially introduced in 2009, SNIP underwent revisions in 2012 to include:
P: Total publications of a source over the last 3 years.
RIP: Raw Impact Per Publication, mirroring the traditional JIF but without field-specific corrections.

% Self-citations: Identifying the proportion of citations that a journal receives from its own publications.

How SNIP Stands Out?

Available on the Scopus citation indexing database by Elsevier, SNIP offers several distinct advantages:

- *Free accessibility*: Even without a Scopus subscription, anyone can access the SNIP rankings.
- *Broad coverage*: SNIP ranks a more extensive range of journals than many other metrics and spans all academic disciplines.

Source Normalized Impact per Paper calculation: To break it down, SNIP is determined by dividing the number of citations in the current year to works published in the previous 3 years by the total publications from the same period. For instance, a SNIP score of 1.0 indicates that a journal has a median citation rate for its field. The uniqueness of SNIP lies in its method of normalization, taking into account the length of the reference list of the citing publication. The longer this list, the lesser the value of the given citation.

Source Normalized Impact per Paper has proven itself as an invaluable tool for academics and researchers. It offers a nuanced understanding of a journal's impact, ensuring a fair comparison across diverse fields. By capturing the essence of a journal's influence in its domain, SNIP simplifies the intricate world of journal metrics.[13]

WHAT ARE ARTICLE-LEVEL METRICS?

Article-level metrics dive deeper than traditional metrics. Instead of evaluating the whole journal's influence, ALMs measure the impact of individual scholarly articles. By looking at both traditional bibliometrics and modern altmetrics, scholars, departments, and administrators gain a clearer picture of an article's influence and reach.

- *Traditional bibliometrics: Citation counts*: At the heart of traditional bibliometrics is the citation count—a straightforward number representing how often an article has been cited by others.
  - *Citation counting overview*:
    - Tells us how many times an article is referenced in other works.
    - Varies based on the database source; for instance, Web of Science might show a different count than Scopus.

    Google Scholar boasts comprehensive coverage but includes references from a wide range of sources, not just high-impact journals.
- *Altmetrics—beyond citations*: Altmetrics represent the digital age's answer to measuring scholarly impact. They encapsulate how research is being shared, discussed, and used in the online realm.
  - *Understanding altmetrics*:
    - Not a replacement for traditional metrics but a complement
    - Offers insights into online activity such as views, downloads, and social media interactions
    - Data is more immediately available than traditional citation counts.
  - *Key altmetric tools*:
    - *Altmetric*: Tracks attention from various online sources, from policy documents and mainstream media to social media platforms like Twitter; aggregates data into an "Attention Score", represented by a colorful donut badge; requires a DOI and compliant metadata for tracking
    - *PlumX metrics*: Breaks down altmetric data into five categories: citations, usage, captures, mentions, and social media; available on many databases and journal webpages

- *The role and significance of ALMs*:
  - *Quick insights*: ALMs provide rapid feedback on an article's impact, especially through altmetrics.
  - *Comprehensive analysis*: By combining bibliometrics and altmetrics, researchers can get a more holistic view of their work's influence.
  - *Flexibility*: ALMs can adapt to the ever-evolving digital landscape, capturing newer forms of scholarly engagement.
- *Caveats and considerations*: While ALMs offer a robust method for assessing scholarly impact, it is crucial to remember:
  - Citation counts and metrics may vary based on the database.
  - ALMs should complement, not replace, peer review and personal impact statements.
  - Statistical interpretation of bibliometrics requires an understanding of underlying assumptions.

Article-level metrics offer a nuanced and comprehensive view of scholarly influence in both traditional and digital spaces. By leveraging both bibliometrics and altmetrics, researchers, academics, and institutions can better understand and communicate the impact of their work in the broader academic community.[13]

AUTHOR-LEVEL METRICS

Author-level metrics are citations metrics that measure the bibliometric impact of individual authors, researchers, academics, and scholars. The most common metric used is *h*-index.

h-INDEX

The *h*-index measures both the productivity and citation impact of a researcher's publications. An *h*-index of 20 means the researcher has 20 papers each cited at least 20 times. This metric is beneficial for evaluating a researcher's overall influence and is particularly pertinent in academic promotions and grant applications.

The *h*-index, introduced by JE Hirsch, serves as a tool to quantify an individual's scientific research output. This metric attempts to balance the productivity (number of articles published) and impact (number of citations) of a researcher's work. Essentially, it offers a snapshot of a scholar's influential contributions to their field of study.

Understanding the *h*-index

To put it simply, if a researcher has an *h*-index of "*n*", they have published "*n*" papers, each of which has been cited in other works at least "*n*" times. However, their additional publications have received fewer than "*n*" citations.

For instance, if Dr Smith has an *h*-index of 7, this indicates that she has published seven papers, each cited at least seven times, but her subsequent papers have been cited fewer than seven times.

Why is *h*-index Important?

- *Balanced measurement*: Unlike other metrics, the *h*-index provides a more comprehensive view by considering both the volume of publications and the number of citations they receive.
- *Mitigates outliers*: A single highly cited publication can skew metrics, but the *h*-index helps neutralize the effect of such anomalies.
- *Consistent growth*: It rewards consistent research contributions over time rather than a one-off successful publication.

Calculating Your *h*-index

While the *h*-index concept is straightforward, its value can vary based on the database used due to the difference in their citation data coverage. Here is how to find it in some popular databases:

- *Scopus*:
    - Conduct an author search
    - Select the author's name to view their publications, citations, and *h*-index
- *Google Scholar*:
    - Set up a Google Scholar citations profile
    - Ensure all the author's publications are listed
- *Web of Science*:
    - Generate a citation report of the author's publications; the *h*-index will be displayed.
    - It is vital to understand that databases might provide varying *h*-index values because they index different journals and have different coverage years.

In **Table 1**, the *h*-index is 8, as the 8th publication has been cited at least eight times, but the 9th has not been cited nine times.

TABLE 1: *h*-index calculation using number of citations.

Publication rank	Number of citations	Cumulative count
1	112	1
2	76	2
3	41	3
4	39	4
5	16	5
6	14	6
7	10	7
8	9	8
9	8	9
–	–	–

The *h*-index offers an insightful metric for evaluating a researcher's impact, but it is essential to view it in conjunction with other metrics to get a comprehensive understanding of a researcher's influence in their field.[14]

HOW TO USE METRICS WISELY?

Selecting journals for publication: When deciding where to publish, a combination of metrics and goals can help guide your choice. These metrics should align with personal and professional aspirations, the objectives of the research, and the desired readership. Beyond mere numbers, consider the broader context of the journal. Factors such as the journal's scope, the review process, the average duration to publication, and the availability of open access options can play pivotal roles in your decision.

Assessing the quality of research: Relying exclusively on journal metrics, like IF, to gauge the quality of research can be misleading; instead, a more holistic approach is recommended.

For a well-rounded evaluation:

- *Complementary evaluation*: It is beneficial to read major articles in your field. This approach ensures you grasp the core ideas without getting blinded by journal metrics.
- *Metrics as a guideline*: While metrics can help point out significant journals in your area, delving into the articles themselves provides a direct assessment of their relevance and quality.

LIMITATIONS AND CRITICISMS OF JOURNAL METRICS

Concerns with Impact Factor

- *Misuse*: The IF is often erroneously used as an indicator of the quality of individual articles. However, it was never intended for such granular evaluation.
- *Inflation tactics*: Some journals might encourage authors to cite papers from the same journal, a tactic that can artificially boost the IF.

General Concerns

- *Language and geographical bias*: Journals that are not in English or those that do not belong to the dominant Western scientific community may not be adequately represented in metrics.
- *Overlooking innovation*: A high metric score does not necessarily correlate with pioneering or innovative research.

LOOKING AHEAD: FUTURE OF JOURNAL METRICS

Emergence of New Metrics

- *Altmetrics*: These capture the online footprint of research. By tracking mentions on social media, blog discussions, and other online platforms, altmetrics give a more comprehensive picture of how the research is being received and discussed beyond academic circles.
- *Usage metrics*: These metrics, including article views and downloads, offer real-time feedback on the level of interest a research piece garners.
- *Holistic approaches*: In the future, it is anticipated that there will be a shift toward integrating both traditional and novel metrics. This blend will offer a more comprehensive view of a journal's influence and the wider impact of research. Such an approach acknowledges the multifaceted nature of research impact, recognizing both academic citations and broader societal engagement.

The landscape of journal metrics is rapidly evolving. Journal metrics are valuable tools, offering objective data to guide decision-making for medical postgraduates. However, their application requires careful consideration, contextual understanding, and awareness of their limitations. As the academic landscape evolves, so too will these metrics and their interpretations, necessitating ongoing engagement and learning within the medical scholarly community.

CONCLUSION

In the dynamic world of academic publishing, understanding and leveraging journal metrics is of paramount importance. As we have journeyed through this chapter, it is evident that while metrics like IF provide a snapshot of a journal's influence, they are just a part of a much larger, complex picture. A holistic approach, integrating both traditional metrics and emerging ones like altmetrics, is essential to truly grasp the breadth and depth of a research piece's impact. Furthermore, while metrics can guide decisions and provide insight, they should be used judiciously, complemented by a researcher's own informed judgment. As academia continues to evolve with the digital age, it is crucial for researchers to stay updated, adaptable, and critical in their approach to journal metrics.

REFERENCES

1. Tregoning J. How will you judge me if not by impact factor? Nature. 2018;558(7710):345.
2. Chavda J, Patel A. Measuring research impact: bibliometrics, social media, altmetrics, and the BJGP. Br J Gen Pract. 2016;66(642):e59-61.
3. Boudry C, Chartron G. Availability of digital object identifiers in publications archived by PubMed. Scientometrics. 2017;110(3):1453-69.

4. Eldakar MAM. Who reads international Egyptian academic articles? An altmetrics analysis of Mendeley readership categories. Scientometrics. 2019;121(1):105-35.
5. Gasparyan AY, Yessirkepov M, Voronov AA, Maksaev AA, Kitas GD. Article-Level Metrics. J Korean Med Sci. 2021;36(11):e74.
6. Garfield E. Citation indexes for science; a new dimension in documentation through association of ideas. Science. 1955;122 (3159):108-11.
7. Garfield E. "Science Citation Index"–A new dimension in indexing. Science. 1964; 144(3619):649-54.
8. Margolis J. Citation indexing and evaluation of scientific papers. Science. 1967;155(3767): 1213-9.
9. Price DJ. Networks of scientific papers. Science. 1965;149(3683):510-5.
10. Ali MJ. Questioning the Impact of the Impact Factor. A Brief Review and Future Directions. Semin Ophthalmol. 2022;37(1):91-6.
11. Falagas ME, Kouranos VD, Arencibia-Jorge R, Karageorgopoulos DE. Comparison of SCImago journal rank indicator with journal impact factor. Faseb J. 2008;22:2623-8.
12. University of Maryland. (2023). Bibliometrics and Altmetrics: Measuring the Impact of Knowledge. [online] Available from https://lib.guides.umd.edu/bibliometrics/altmetrics [Last accessed January, 2024].
13. Daemen Library. (2023). Research Impact and Scholarly Metrics. [online] Available from https://libguides.daemen.edu/c.php?g=1239513&p=9071368 [Last accessed January, 2024].
14. Shah FA, Jawaid SA. The *h*-Index: An Indicator of Research and Publication Output. Pak J Med Sci. 2023;39(2):315-6.

CHAPTER 14

How to Submit a Manuscript?

Shambo Samrat Samajdar

INTRODUCTION

As medical professionals, you dedicate your time and expertise to advancing healthcare through research and innovation. One crucial aspect of this journey is sharing your findings with the broader scientific community, and a common avenue for doing so is by submitting your manuscript to a reputable medical journal. However, the process of manuscript submission can often seem daunting, with each journal having its own unique set of requirements and guidelines. In this chapter, we will delve into the essential steps and considerations for successfully submitting your medical manuscript to a journal.

GET FAMILIAR WITH THE JOURNAL'S INSTRUCTIONS FOR AUTHORS

Before embarking on your manuscript submission journey, it is imperative to acquaint yourself with the journal's "instructions for authors" (IFAs). These instructions are not a mere formality but a roadmap that guides potential authors on how to construct their articles correctly and prepare them for submission. They are, in essence, the keys to unlock the doors to publication in your chosen journal.[1]

Understanding the Journal's Individual Requirements

Instructions for authors are not one-size-fits-all; they are tailored to each journal's specific needs and expectations. They tell you precisely what the journal's editorial board anticipates seeing in your submission.[1] These guidelines encompass more than just the format of your manuscript; they also provide insight into the journal's unique processes and requirements that, if followed meticulously, can help ensure a smooth journey from submission to publication.

What Information is Included in the Instructions for Authors?

The IFAs comprise a comprehensive repository of information critical to your manuscript's success. Within their pages, you will find:

- *Information about the journal*: This section will enlighten you about the journal's scope, the types of articles it accepts, the preferred language for publication, and other key insights that will help you determine if the journal is the right fit for your research.[2]
- *Article preparation requirements*: These guidelines encompass essential details such as word count restrictions, style guides, and specific formatting instructions. You will also discover if the journal provides article templates that can be used as a starting point for your manuscript.
- *Manuscript submission process*: Here, you will learn about the technical aspects of submitting your work, including which online submission system the journal employs. Understanding this process is crucial to ensure your manuscript reaches the right hands efficiently.
- *Specific policies and procedures*: Many medical journals have specific policies regarding clinical trial registration, ethics compliance, and other important aspects. Familiarizing yourself with these policies is essential to avoid potential pitfalls during the submission and review process.[1]
- *Your publishing options*: Lastly, the IFAs may provide information on publishing options, including the possibility of open-access publication. This section will help you make informed decisions about how you want your work to be disseminated.[2]

NAVIGATING THE JOURNAL SELECTION MAZE: FINDING THE PERFECT FIT FOR YOUR MANUSCRIPT

Selecting the right journal for your manuscript is akin to laying the foundation for a successful publication journey. This pivotal decision, often underestimated, holds the power to determine whether your research finds its deserved spotlight or languishes in obscurity. When embarking on this critical step, consider an array of factors that can significantly impact your manuscript's acceptance and visibility.

Understanding the Journal's Audience and Scope

A fundamental consideration is the journal's target audience. Assess the breadth of your research's implications and determine whether it might appeal to researchers across various fields or is more tailored to a specific niche. Opt for a journal whose readership aligns with your research goals to maximize its reach and impact. A glance at the journal's previously published articles can provide valuable insights into the topics that capture the editors' interest.[2]

Matching Research Focus with Journal Aims

Delve into the aims and scope of the journal to ensure it aligns with your research focus. Whether your work is applied, clinical, or basic research, there is a journal out there tailored to your needs. Take time to investigate the types of articles the journal typically publishes, especially if you are planning a *review article* or a specialized contribution. Additionally, check if the journal imposes any length restrictions and whether your manuscript can comfortably comply.

Beyond Impact Factor: Reputation and Indexing

While a journal's *impact factor* can be alluring, it is not the sole indicator of its prestige. Delve deeper by examining the caliber of authors who publish in the journal and whether it enjoys recognition within your specific field. Equally important is the journal's presence in indexing sites and databases like PubMed, Scopus, or Web of Science. Ensure that your chosen journal's indexing aligns with the platforms your peers use to discover relevant research.[2,3]

Compliance with Funding Mandates

In an era of increasing open access mandates from funding bodies, its crucial to verify whether your selected journal's policies allow you to comply with these requirements. Explore options for making your research open access, whether through repository deposit or open-access publication, and ensure the journal facilitates this.[4]

As you embark on the journey of manuscript submission, the strategic selection of the right journal should be a well-considered step. Start this process after accumulating sufficient research results but before diving into manuscript composition. Begin with journals encountered during your literature review, and do not overlook the treasure trove of suitable outlets hidden within the references of papers you have read. By carefully navigating the journal selection maze, you pave the way for your research to shine on the global academic stage.

STRATEGIC JOURNAL SELECTION: NAVIGATING TOWARD THE PERFECT MATCH

Once you have compiled a list of potential journals for your manuscript, the next step is to dig deeper into each one. Visit the websites of these journals and seek out their dedicated "instructions for authors" sections. Here, you will find a treasure trove of vital information, including guidelines on manuscript preparation and submission, which further refine your choices based on the factors discussed earlier. As you explore these guidelines, journals that do not align with your manuscript's focus, audience, or your publication goals should be swiftly eliminated from consideration. Among the remaining contenders, there is likely to be one or more that shine as excellent candidates. At this juncture, consider whether conducting additional experiments or refining certain aspects of your study could enhance your chances of publication in your top choice. If speed is of the essence, investigate which of the remaining journals offers rapid publication, or assess their publication frequency if time is a constraint. For those aiming to maximize readership, seriously contemplate journals that offer an open-access option. Open access ensures that your research is readily accessible to all, fostering greater visibility and potential for citation.[1,4]

Furthermore, it is prudent to identify not just your first-choice journal but also second and third choices. This preemptive planning allows for a seamless transition should your manuscript be rejected by your primary target. Many publishers now facilitate manuscript transfers between journals within their portfolio, sparing you from reformatting and in some cases, even preserving reviewer reports from the initial submission. Keep an eye out for journals that participate in such transfer schemes, as they make for excellent backup options. In this intricate dance of journal selection, meticulous planning can be the key to a successful manuscript submission journey.

MEETING THE EDITOR'S EXPECTATIONS: KEY FACTORS FOR MANUSCRIPT ACCEPTANCE

Understanding what journal editors seek in a manuscript is pivotal to increasing your chances of publication success. Editors play a crucial role in evaluating and selecting manuscripts for publication, and their decisions often hinge on several critical factors. Editors operate under tight schedules, requiring them to quickly assess a submission's suitability. When presented with a manuscript, they typically first scrutinize the cover letter, abstract, conclusion, and references. These components serve as initial touchpoints to determine if the submission aligns with the journal's scope and possesses sufficient impact.[5] In essence, journal editors strive to balance the novelty and significance of a paper with the expectations of their readership and the journal's overall impact. Their ultimate goal is to publish high-quality science that captivates and benefits their audience. To maximize your manuscript's chances of acceptance, it is imperative to ensure that it:

- *Falls within the journal's scope*: A manuscript should fit seamlessly within the journal's subject matter.
- *Presents novel research*: Editors seek work that advances the field and offers fresh insights.

- *Contributes to an active research area*: Manuscripts that engage with and build upon ongoing scientific discussions often find favor.
- *Is meticulously prepared*: Proper formatting and inclusion of all required sections demonstrate professionalism.
- *Communicates clearly*: Clarity and conciseness in language and presentation are highly valued.
- *Adheres to ethical standards*: Editors prioritize research that upholds ethical guidelines and practices.

Ultimately, your manuscript should convey a scientific message that underscores the study's significance. A valuable tip is to have a colleague review your manuscript for flow and impact, making any necessary revisions to ensure it captures the editor's attention. By aligning your work with the editor's expectations, you enhance your manuscript's prospects of making its mark in the world of scientific publication.

CRAFTING AN EFFECTIVE COVER LETTER: YOUR MANUSCRIPT'S FIRST IMPRESSION

A well-structured and persuasive cover letter serves as your manuscript's introduction to the journal editor. It is not just a formality; it is your opportunity to make a compelling case for why your work deserves a place in the journal's pages. While writing your cover letter, it is essential to adhere to any specific requirements outlined in the journal's IFAs. Tailoring your letter to the editor's expectations can significantly enhance your chances of success.

Begin by addressing the editor by name if known, followed by the date of submission and the journal to which you are applying. The first paragraph should succinctly introduce your manuscript, including its title and type (e.g., research, review, case study). Here, briefly outline the study's background, the question you aimed to answer, and the rationale behind your research.

In the second paragraph, provide a concise summary of your methods, main findings, and their significance. Editors appreciate clarity and brevity, so present your work's essence effectively.

The third paragraph is a crucial opportunity to explain why the journal's readers would find your work compelling. Align your study with the journal's aims and scope, highlighting its broad implications if required. Emphasize the importance of your results to the field, demonstrating how your research contributes to the ongoing discourse.

Conclude your cover letter by specifying the corresponding author and addressing any journal-specific requirements, such as ethical standards. Two essential sentences that should always be included affirm that the manuscript has not been published elsewhere and is not under consideration by another journal. Confirm that all authors have approved the manuscript's submission to the target journal.

Before final submission, meticulously review your manuscript to ensure it adheres to the IFAs, complies with file format and quality standards, and is free from spelling and grammar errors. Do not underestimate the power of a persuasive cover letter—it is your manuscript's first impression, and a well-crafted one can significantly bolster your chances of successful publication.

SUBMISSION SUCCESS: A CHECKLIST BEFORE YOU HIT "SUBMIT"

Submitting your manuscript to a journal is the culmination of your hard work and dedication to your research. However, before you take that final step and send your work out into the world, it is crucial to perform a thorough quality check to ensure everything is in order. Consider this your last chance to fine-tune your submission and maximize your chances of acceptance.

Begin by verifying that your manuscript meticulously adheres to the journal's IFAs. These guidelines are your roadmap to ensuring your work aligns with the journal's requirements and standards. Next, take a close look at the technical aspects of your submission. Ensure that all files are in the correct file format and meet the journal's specifications for resolution and size. Mistakes in file formatting can lead to unnecessary delays or complications during the review process. A critical review of your manuscript's language and presentation is equally essential. Check for spelling and grammar errors that could detract from the professionalism and readability of your work. Additionally, confirm that you have up-to-date contact information for all authors. Accurate contact details are vital for effective communication during the submission and review process. Lastly, revisit your cover letter. Ensure that it is not only well-written but also persuasive. A compelling cover letter serves as your manuscript's ambassador, making a strong case for its inclusion in the journal.

By diligently completing this submission checklist, you not only enhance the quality of your manuscript but also streamline the submission process. Attention to detail at this stage can make the difference between a smooth journey toward publication and potential setbacks.

PEER REVIEW PROCESS: ELEVATING YOUR MANUSCRIPT TO EXCELLENCE

The peer review process, a cornerstone of scholarly publishing, can evoke mixed emotions in authors. It serves as the gatekeeper that ensures scientific journals disseminate high-quality research beneficial to the wider scientific community. While the prospect of manuscript rejection might appear daunting, it is crucial to view peer review as a constructive and positive mechanism that ultimately enhances the quality and impact of your work. Peer review engages experts within your field who voluntarily dedicate their time to evaluate and improve the manuscripts they review, providing authors with invaluable insights and feedback at no cost. This collaborative effort aims to refine your research on multiple fronts.

Firstly, peer reviewers act as a diligent second set of eyes, identifying any gaps in your study that may necessitate additional explanations or supplementary experiments. This critical examination strengthens the scientific rigor of your work, ensuring that it withstands scrutiny. Secondly, reviewers assess the clarity and comprehensibility of your manuscript. They pinpoint areas that might be challenging to grasp, prompting you to revise and enhance the clarity of your presentation. After all, if experts struggle to understand your research, it is unlikely to resonate with readers from diverse backgrounds. Moreover, peer reviewers evaluate the significance of your paper within the context of your field. They offer suggestions to amplify its impact, making it more valuable and relevant to researchers and readers alike.

Significantly, the peer review process acts as a quality control measure. It ensures that the manuscripts published in a journal align with the journal's specific aims and meet the high standards expected within the scientific community.

Embrace the peer review process as an opportunity for growth and refinement. It is a pathway to elevating the impact of your research and contributing meaningfully to the advancement of science. Through collaboration and constructive feedback, your manuscript undergoes a transformation, emerging as a more robust, comprehensible, and impactful piece of scientific work. **Table 1** describes different types of peer review process.

TABLE 1: Types of peer review process.

Single anonymized	Author does not know the identity of the reviewer
Double anonymized	Reviewer does not know the identity of the author, and vice versa
Open peer review	The identity of the author and the reviewer is known by all participants, during or after the review process
Transparent peer review	Review report is posted with the published article. Reviewer can choose if they want to share their identity
Collaborative	Two or more reviewers work together to submit a unified report OR Author revises manuscript under the supervision of one or more reviewers
Post publication	Review solicited or unsolicited, of a published paper and does not exclude other forms of peer review (not significant for this discussion)

UNDERSTANDING AND ADDRESSING MANUSCRIPT REJECTIONS: TECHNICAL AND EDITORIAL ASPECTS

The journey of submitting a manuscript to a journal can sometimes be fraught with the disappointment of rejection. To effectively navigate this process, it is crucial to grasp the common reasons manuscripts face rejection, which typically fall into two categories: technical and editorial.

Technical Reasons for Rejection

These issues often require additional work before your manuscript can meet the journal's standards for publication. They encompass:

- *Incomplete data*: Manuscripts may be rejected if they have inadequate data, such as a small sample size or missing and poorly executed controls.
- *Poor analysis*: Using inappropriate statistical tests or failing to include statistical analysis can lead to rejection.
- *Inappropriate methodology*: Outdated or unsuitable methods for addressing your research question may result in rejection. Modern, more robust methodologies are often preferred.
- *Weak research motive*: Manuscripts may be rejected if the hypothesis is unclear, scientifically invalid, or if the data fails to address the research question effectively.
- *Inaccurate conclusions*: Drawing conclusions that are not supported by your data can lead to rejection. It is vital to base your conclusions on the evidence presented.

Editorial Reasons for Rejection

These reasons pertain to the manuscript's overall fit and ethical considerations, including:

- *Out of scope*: Manuscripts may be rejected if they do not align with the journal's scope and subject matter.
- *Lack of significance*: If the research is not deemed a significant advancement within the field, it might face rejection.
- *Ethical concerns*: Manuscripts lacking proper ethical approvals, such as patient consent or ethics committee approval for animal research, can be rejected.
- *Structural issues*: Manuscripts that do not adhere to the journal's formatting and structural requirements may be rejected.
- *Lack of detail*: Inadequate information to understand and replicate the analysis and experiments can lead to rejection.
- *Reference quality*: Overreliance on self-citations or outdated references may result in rejection.
- *Language quality*: Manuscripts with poor language quality that hinder reader comprehension may face rejection.

- *Logical coherence*: Difficult-to-follow logic or poorly presented data can be grounds for rejection.
- *Ethical violations*: Violations of publication ethics, such as plagiarism or data manipulation, can lead to rejection.

To minimize the chances of rejection, invest time in comprehensive research, hypothesis development, and experiment planning. Follow the journal's specific guidelines, craft a coherent and well-written paper, and perform an honest assessment of your work when selecting a target journal. By addressing these technical and editorial considerations, you can enhance the quality and readiness of your manuscript for successful submission.

NAVIGATING MANUSCRIPT REVISIONS AND RESPONDING TO PEER REVIEW

Receiving feedback from reviewers is a pivotal moment in the publication journey, offering the opportunity to refine your manuscript and address any concerns raised by experts in the field. Typically, you will receive a letter from the editor who handled your manuscript, detailing the revisions required and providing access to the reviewer reports. This letter also outlines the process for returning your revised manuscript, including instructions on how to highlight the changes made and the submission deadline. It is essential to be mindful of varying revision deadlines set by different journals, ranging from a few weeks to several months, depending on the extent of revisions needed. If you anticipate challenges in meeting the deadline, promptly communicate with the editor to discuss the possibility of an extension.[5]

When revising your manuscript and responding to peer review comments, adhere to a structured approach:[6]

- *Express gratitude*: Begin by thanking the reviewers and editors for their time and valuable feedback. A courteous tone sets a positive tone for the revision process.
- *Comprehensive response*: Address all points raised by the editor and reviewers, demonstrating your commitment to improving the manuscript.
- *Major revisions*: Clearly describe the major revisions made to your manuscript in your response letter. Follow this with a point-by-point response to the comments raised, providing detailed explanations and justifications for your changes.
- *Additional experiments or analyses*: If reviewers recommend additional experiments or analyses, consider their suggestions seriously. Undertake these unless you can justify why they would not enhance your paper, and explain your reasoning in your response letter.
- *Scientific rebuttal*: If you disagree with specific points or comments, offer a polite and scientific rebuttal in your response letter. Keep in mind that this letter may be seen by subsequent reviewers if your manuscript undergoes a second round of peer review.

- *Differentiation*: Clearly distinguish between reviewer comments and your responses in your letter for clarity.
- *Highlight revisions*: Make it easy for reviewers to identify the changes in your manuscript. Use different text colors, highlight alterations, or employ word processing tools like Microsoft Word's Track Changes feature. This visual aid complements your written explanations.
- *Timely submission*: Ensure that you return the revised manuscript and response letter within the specified timeframe outlined by the editor.

Responding to reviewer comments is a critical phase where effective communication, transparency, and respect for differing opinions are paramount. Whether you agree or disagree with reviewers, maintaining a professional and courteous demeanor in your responses fosters a constructive dialogue that ultimately benefits your manuscript's quality and its journey toward publication.

NAVIGATING MANUSCRIPT REJECTIONS: WHEN TO CONSIDER AN APPEAL

Experiencing a manuscript rejection can be disheartening, but it is essential to discern when it is appropriate to contest a decision and when it is wiser to seek publication elsewhere. When faced with rejection, it is advisable to take a few days to carefully consider your options before deciding your next steps.

It is worth noting that appeals of rejection decisions are rarely successful and tend to be approved only in exceptional cases. Success typically hinges on your ability to provide robust evidence or new data that can address and alleviate the concerns expressed by the editor and reviewers. It is important to approach appeals rationally rather than emotionally, as they are subject to journal policies and given lower priority than new submissions. Resolving appeals may take several weeks, if not longer.

If you choose to proceed with an appeal letter, follow these guidelines:[5-8]

- *Clear explanation*: Clearly articulate why you disagree with the decision and present any new information that you believe should be taken into account. Avoid repetition of content from your original submission or cover letter.
- *Addressing shortcomings*: If editors or reviewers have highlighted shortcomings in your paper that you can address, outline how you intend to do so, including providing additional data if necessary.
- *Point-by-point response*: Provide a systematic, point-by-point response to any reviewer comments, demonstrating your commitment to addressing their concerns.
- *Evidence-based arguments*: If you believe that a reviewer has made technical errors in their assessment or displayed bias, substantiate your opinion with evidence.

- Importantly, avoid personal attacks on the editors or reviewers in your appeal. Editorial decisions are multifaceted, and one rejection does not necessarily preclude future consideration of your work by the same journal or editor.

Typically, journals accept only one letter defending your submission for each of the review stages (editorial review and peer review).[9] If your response is unsuccessful after sending such a letter, it is prudent to seriously consider submitting your work to another journal. In certain situations, you may find it necessary to submit your manuscript to another journal before receiving a decision, especially if your results are time-sensitive or if the review process is significantly delayed. In such cases, it is essential to formally withdraw your manuscript from the initial journal and obtain confirmation of the withdrawal before submitting it elsewhere. This courteous approach ensures transparency and professionalism in the publishing process.

CONCLUSION: THE MANUSCRIPT JOURNEY—FROM SUBMISSION TO CELEBRATION

The process of submitting a manuscript to a journal is a significant undertaking, often marked by dedication, perseverance, and scholarly rigor. As we conclude this chapter on how to submit a manuscript in a journal, it is important to reflect on the journey and acknowledge the key milestones that lead to publication.

- *Celebrate your achievement*: The journey from drafting your research to navigating the intricate world of peer review and revisions is no small feat. When you receive that long-awaited acceptance notification, take a moment to celebrate. You have crossed a significant milestone in your academic and scientific career.
- *The final steps*: As you near the finish line, there are two crucial final steps to consider. First, review the "proof"—a PDF version that offers an exact preview of how your article will look once published. This meticulous review ensures that your work is presented accurately and professionally.
- *Embrace digital publication*: With the advent of digital publishing, your work can reach a global audience with ease. Once the "prepress" version, identical to the printed article, is available online, seize the opportunity to share your research with the world. If your journal permits, use social media platforms and your own website to publicize your article. This step not only broadens your research's reach but also contributes to the dissemination of knowledge within your field.
- *Lessons from experience*: The journey of publishing research often comes with moments of reflection. As Andrew R Schrock aptly notes, minor grammatical errors can linger as reminders of late-night editing sessions. These experiences teach us the importance of attentiveness, patience, and the recognition that perfection is a journey, not a destination.

In the world of academic publishing, every manuscript submitted is a step toward advancing human knowledge. It is a testament to your dedication to the pursuit of truth and the betterment of society. So, as you embark on your manuscript submission journey, remember the collective progress that stems from every researcher's contribution, and may your scholarly endeavors continue to illuminate the path of discovery for generations to come.

REFERENCES

1. Editorials, Springer Nature Limited. (2020). Communication is key to constructive peer review. [online] Available from media.nature.com/original/magazine-assets/d41586-020-01622-z/d41586-020-01622-z.pdf [Last accessed January, 2024].
2. Elmore SA, Weston EH. Predatory journals: what they are and how to avoid them. Toxicol Pathol. 2020;48(4):607-10.
3. Goodman SN, Berlin S, Fletcher SW, Fletcher RH. Manuscript quality before and after peer review and editing at Annals of Internal Medicine. Ann Intern Med. 1994;121:11-21.
4. Hall GM. How to Write a Paper, 5th edition. Chichester, West Sussex, UK: Wiley-Blackwell; 2013.
5. Gray T. Publish and Flourish: Become a Prolific Scholar, 15th anniversary edition. Las Cruces: Teaching Academy, New Mexico State University; 2020.
6. Halm EA, Landon BE. (2007). Everything you wanted to know about writing a research abstract but were too afraid (or started too late) to ask. [online] Available from www.sgim.org/File%20Library/SGIM/Resource%20Library/Forum/2007/Forum200712.pdf [Last accessed January, 2024].
7. Hancock E. Ideas into Words: Mastering the Craft of Science Writing. Baltimore: Johns Hopkins University Press; 2003.
8. Huth EJ. Medical Style and Format: An International Manual for Authors, Editors, and Publishers. Baltimore: Williams and Wilkins; 1987.
9. International Committee of Medical Journal Editors. (2019). Recommendations for the conduct, reporting, editing, and publication of scholarly work in medical journals. [online] Available from www.icmje.org/icmje-recommendations.pdf [Last accessed January, 2024].

CHAPTER 15

Fee Structure

Shambo Samrat Samajdar

INTRODUCTION

The importance of understanding publication fees: In the realm of scientific publication, the landscape has evolved significantly in recent years. One crucial aspect of this transformation is the advent of article processing charges (APCs), often referred to as publishing fees. These charges are becoming increasingly prevalent and can have a profound impact on how research is disseminated. Therefore, as aspiring authors and early-career researchers, it is paramount that you grasp the intricacies of publication fees and their implications. Publishing fees, in essence, are the financial costs associated with getting your research findings into the hands of your peers and the wider academic community. They are a vital component of the broader discourse on open access, a movement advocating for unrestricted access to scholarly work. Understanding these fees is not just a matter of financial literacy, it is an essential skill that empowers you to make informed decisions about where and how you publish your research.[1]

How fees vary across different types of publications?: The world of academic publishing is diverse, with a multitude of journals and publishers, each operating under distinct models and fee structures. As you embark on your journey into the world of scientific publication, you will encounter various types of publication fees. From APCs to submission fees, page charges, and open-access fees, the choices can be bewildering. It is crucial to comprehend the differences among these fees, what they cover, and when and why they apply. Notably, not all journals and publishers require the same fees, and the amount you might be expected to pay can vary significantly. This chapter will shed light on the different fee models and help you navigate this complex terrain with confidence.[1,2]

The impact of fees on your research and budget: The decisions you make regarding publication fees can have far-reaching consequences for your research, your academic career, and your budget. It is not merely a matter of writing a paper, submitting it, and seeing it published. The financial aspects of publishing can influence your ability to disseminate your work, the quality of the journal you choose, and the accessibility of your research to others.[2] Moreover, understanding the financial implications of publication fees is essential for budgeting your research endeavors effectively. With the rising costs associated with academic publishing, being prepared and informed about these expenses is paramount for researchers, especially those operating within financially constrained institutions or as students.

In this chapter, we will explore the intricacies of publication fees, the various types of charges you may encounter, and how to navigate this terrain to ensure your research reaches its full potential. By the end of this chapter, you will be better equipped to make informed decisions about where and how to publish your scientific work, taking into consideration the financial aspects that can shape the trajectory of your research career.

TYPES OF PUBLICATION FEES[3]

Article Processing Charges

Definition and explanation: APCs are fees imposed on authors or their institutions to cover the costs associated with the publication of their research papers. These charges are commonly associated with open-access journals and are intended to ensure that research articles are freely accessible to the public.

Examples of journals using APCs: Notable examples of journals using APCs include PLOS ONE, Frontiers in Psychology, and BioMed Central (BMC) series.

Factors affecting APCs: APCs can vary widely, ranging from a few hundred dollars to several thousand dollars per article. Factors influencing the cost of APCs include the journal's reputation, impact factor, the publisher's pricing policy, the length of the article, and the type of open-access license chosen by the author.

Submission Fees

What submission fees are and when they apply?: Submission fees are charges levied on authors at the time of manuscript submission to a journal, before the peer review process begins. These fees are distinct from publication fees and are intended to cover the administrative costs associated with managing the submission process.

How submission fees differ from publication fees?: Submission fees are paid upfront when submitting a manuscript, whereas publication fees are paid after the manuscript has been accepted for publication. Submission fees are nonrefundable and do not guarantee acceptance of the manuscript.

Reasons for submission fees: Submission fees help journals manage the volume of incoming manuscripts by discouraging low-quality or inappropriate submissions.

They also offset the costs of manuscript processing, initial screening, and administrative tasks related to submissions.[4]

Page Charges

Explanation of page charges: Page charges are fees associated with the publication of printed articles in traditional academic journals. Authors are billed based on the number of pages their articles occupy in the print version of the journal.

Journals and publishers using page charges: Many traditional subscription-based journals, particularly in scientific and technical fields, impose page charges. These charges are less common in open-access journals, as they primarily apply to print publications.

How page charges are calculated?: Page charges are typically calculated based on the number of printed pages occupied by the article, with additional fees for color figures or supplementary materials.

Open-access Fees

What open-access fees cover?: Open-access fees, also known as author publication charges or APCs, cover the costs associated with making research articles freely accessible to the public. These fees support the peer review process, online distribution, and open-access infrastructure.

Benefits of open-access publishing: Open-access publishing ensures that research findings are accessible to a global audience without barriers, increasing the visibility and impact of the research. It fosters collaboration, knowledge dissemination, and innovation by eliminating paywalls.

Exploring hybrid open-access models: Some journals offer hybrid open-access models, where authors can choose to make their articles available in open access for a fee within a subscription-based journal. Hybrid models aim to strike a balance between open-access principles and traditional subscription revenue.[1,4]

Understanding these types of publication fees is essential for researchers and authors, as it enables informed decision-making when selecting the appropriate journal for their research and managing the associated costs effectively.

BUDGETING FOR PUBLICATION FEES

Evaluating Your Research Funding

Before embarking on the publication journey, it is crucial for researchers to assess their available research funding. Consider the following factors:

Research grants: Determine whether you have research grants or funding from institutions, government agencies, or private foundations that can cover publication fees.

Institutional support: Check if your academic institution provides financial support for publishing research, either through departmental funds or institutional repositories.

Researcher funds: Some researchers maintain personal funds or budgets for research-related expenses, including publication fees.

Collaborative funding: If you are collaborating with others on a project, explore whether they have access to funding that can help cover publication costs.[3,4]

Planning for Publication Expenses

Once you have evaluated your research funding, create a comprehensive plan for managing publication expenses:

Identify potential costs: Determine the type of publication fees your chosen journal may require, such as APCs, submission fees, or page charges.

Budget allocation: Allocate a portion of your research budget specifically for publication expenses. Be sure to account for potential variations in fees depending on the journal and publishing model.

Prioritize journals: Consider the prestige and impact factor of journals in your field. Balance the benefits of publishing in high-impact journals with the associated costs.[5]

Explore waiver options: Investigate whether the journal offers fee waivers for authors with financial constraints, and check if you qualify for such waivers.

Strategies for Managing Publication Costs

To effectively manage publication costs, implement the following strategies:

Open-access journals: Explore open-access journals, which may have different fee structures. Some may have lower APCs or offer alternatives like reduced fees for researchers from low-income countries.

Hybrid models: Consider journals that offer hybrid publishing models, allowing you to choose whether to pay for open access or publish traditionally. This flexibility can help control costs.

Membership discounts: Join professional societies or organizations related to your field, as they often offer membership discounts for publishing in affiliated journals.

Timing: Plan your submissions strategically to maximize your research funding. If you have limited funds, prioritize publishing your most impactful work.

Seeking Alternative Funding Sources

In addition to traditional research funding, explore alternative sources to cover publication fees:

Author institutions: Check if your academic institution has agreements with publishers that cover or discount publication fees for affiliated researchers.

Research funders: Some research funders explicitly allocate a portion of their grants for publication fees. Ensure you comply with their guidelines.

Grants for open access: Seek grants specifically designed to support open-access publishing, which can help offset APCs.

Crowdfunding: Consider crowdfunding platforms or research-specific crowd-funding campaigns to raise funds for publication fees.

Collaborative funding: Collaborate with coauthors or colleagues to share the financial burden of publication fees, especially if you are publishing jointly.[6]

By carefully evaluating your research funding, planning for publication expenses, implementing cost-effective strategies, and seeking alternative funding sources, you can navigate the world of publication fees with greater ease and ensure that your valuable research reaches a wider audience.

NEGOTIATING PUBLICATION FEES

When and How to Negotiate Fees?

Negotiating publication fees can be a critical aspect of the publishing process, especially when you are facing financial constraints or considering options to reduce costs. Here is when and how to negotiate fees effectively:

Timing matters: Start thinking about negotiation early in the submission process. While some fees are non-negotiable, others can be discussed at different stages, so be prepared to initiate discussions when appropriate.

Identify eligibility: Determine if you qualify for waivers or discounts based on your affiliation, research funding, or the journal's policies. Many journals offer specific criteria for fee reductions, and it is essential to understand these guidelines.

Contact the journal: Reach out to the journal's editorial or customer service staff to inquire about available options for fee negotiation. Email is often the preferred mode of communication for such inquiries.

Prepare a request: When contacting the journal, be clear and concise in your request. Explain your situation, eligibility for discounts, and reasons for requesting a fee reduction. Provide any necessary documentation to support your case.

Tips for Successful Fee Negotiations

Negotiating publication fees can be more successful with the following tips:

Politeness and professionalism: Maintain a polite and professional tone in all your communication with journal representatives. A courteous approach is more likely to yield positive results.

Highlight benefits: Emphasize the value your research brings to the journal. Explain how your work aligns with the journal's scope and why it is essential for both parties to find a mutually beneficial solution.

Offer collaboration: Sometimes, offering to collaborate with the journal in other ways, such as becoming a reviewer or contributing to their outreach efforts, can strengthen your negotiation position.

Be flexible: Be open to compromises. If the journal cannot offer a full waiver, explore options for partial reductions or deferred payments to make publishing more manageable.

Understanding Waivers and Discounts

Understanding the types of waivers and discounts available can help you navigate negotiations more effectively:

Country-based waivers: Many journals offer waivers or reduced fees based on the World Bank's classification of your country's income level. Low-income or lower-middle-income countries often receive full or partial waivers.

Financial hardship: Journals may consider fee reductions for authors facing financial hardship. Be prepared to provide evidence of your financial situation, such as institutional support limitations or personal financial constraints.

Editorial discretion: In some cases, journals may grant waivers or discounts at the editor's discretion. This typically applies when there is a compelling reason, such as a critical review of a previously published article in the same journal.

Error-related refunds: Some publishers offer refunds if errors on their part lead to publication issues, such as incorrect licensing or accessibility problems. Keep this in mind if you encounter such problems after publication.[6]

In conclusion, negotiating publication fees requires proactive communication, adherence to guidelines, and a willingness to collaborate. Approach negotiations respectfully and professionally, and be prepared to make a strong case for why a waiver or discount is warranted. Understanding the available options and eligibility criteria can significantly impact your success in negotiating publication fees.

ETHICAL CONSIDERATIONS

Avoiding Predatory Publishers and Journals

Ethical considerations play a vital role in the world of scientific publishing, particularly when it comes to selecting publishers and journals. Avoiding predatory publishers and journals is crucial to maintaining the integrity of your research and contributing to the scientific community responsibly. Here's how to navigate this ethical aspect:

Thorough evaluation: Before submitting your research to a journal, thoroughly evaluate the publisher and journal to ensure they uphold ethical standards. Predatory journals often lack rigorous peer review processes and prioritize profit over academic integrity.

Check for red flags: Look for common attributes associated with predatory journals, such as grammatical errors on their website, lack of transparency, and impractical publication schedules. Be cautious if the journal exhibits any of these signs.

Verify journal indexing: Check if the journal is included in reputable databases like MEDLINE or is affiliated with ethical organizations like the Committee on Publication Ethics (COPE) or the Open Access Scholarly Publishers Association (OASPA).

Utilize reliable resources: Leverage-free and reputable resources like ThinkCheckSubmit.org, the Directory of Open Access Journals (DOAJ), and the SCImago Journal Rank (SJR) to evaluate the quality and legitimacy of journals.[7]

Recognizing Hidden or Excessive Fees

Another ethical concern in scientific publishing is the presence of hidden or excessive fees. Authors should be aware of the costs associated with publishing their research and ensure transparency in fee structures. Here is how to address this issue:

Transparent fee structures: Choose journals that provide clear and transparent information about publication costs. Ethical publishers ensure that authors are fully informed about fees before submission.

Beware of unexplained charges: Be cautious of journals that add unexplained charges during the publication process. Hidden fees can lead to unexpected financial burdens for authors.

Assess value for cost: Evaluate whether the publication fees align with the value and services offered by the journal. Excessive fees without commensurate quality should raise ethical concerns.

Negotiate when appropriate: If fees are a concern, consider negotiating with the journal, especially if you have valid reasons for requesting a waiver or reduction.

Importance of Transparency in Fee Structures

Transparency is a fundamental ethical principle in scientific publishing, particularly in fee structures. Journals should maintain transparency in the following ways:

Disclosure of costs: Journals must clearly disclose all costs associated with publishing, including APCs, submission fees, and any additional charges. Authors should be fully aware of these costs before submission.

Consistent pricing: Journals should have consistent and reasonable pricing structures. Excessive or fluctuating fees without justification can be perceived as unethical.

Clear refund policies: Ethical journals should have clear refund policies in case of errors or discrepancies in the publishing process. Authors should not be financially penalized for journal mistakes.

Communication: Maintain open and clear communication with the journal regarding fees, waivers, or discounts. Ethical publishers are willing to address authors' concerns and inquiries regarding costs.

In conclusion, ethical considerations in fee structures involve avoiding predatory publishers, recognizing hidden fees, and advocating for transparency. Authors should prioritize publishing their research in journals that uphold ethical standards and provide clear and fair fee structures. This not only safeguards the integrity of your research but also contributes to the credibility of the scientific community as a whole.

CRITICISM

In the realm of scientific publishing, the financial implications associated with accessing research publications have become a topic of significant scrutiny and criticism. This section explores the key criticisms and concerns surrounding the fee structures in scientific publishing:

- *Shift of financial responsibility*: One of the primary criticisms revolves around the shift of financial responsibility from readers to writers or their respective backers. APCs have led to a distinct set of apprehensions, as the burden of funding publication costs now falls on authors and their affiliated institutions.

- *Incentive for acceptance*: When publishers derive financial gain from the acceptance of papers, there exists a potential incentive to indiscriminately accept all submissions. This financial motivation may compromise the rigorous criteria required for article selection based on quality. One potential solution to mitigate this issue is the implementation of a fee structure for the peer review process itself, rather than relying solely on fees associated with manuscript acceptance.
- *Impact on institutional budgets*: The transition to open-access publishing has raised concerns about the need to modify institutional budgets to include funds for covering article processing expenses. Inadequate funding may limit the capacity to disseminate research findings, potentially excluding certain studies from the public domain.
- *Shift in funding priorities*: Prominent funding organizations, such as the National Institutes of Health and the Wellcome Trust, have faced criticism for shifting financial support from directly sponsoring research to supporting open-access publication. This shift in funding priorities may have implications for the research landscape.
- *Profit margins of publishers*: Publishers have come under scrutiny for their substantial operational profit margins, often derived from publicly funded research efforts. Such profits, as well as copyright practices, have raised ethical concerns. For instance, some publishers have reported profit margins that surpass those of major technology companies like Apple, Google, and Amazon.
- *Unequal access*: The issue of unequal access to publishing is a significant concern, potentially excluding researchers from lower-income countries or less-funded research disciplines due to the absence of discounts or external financing for APCs.
- *Justification of costs*: Some publishers rationalize a portion of the article processing price by attributing it to the expenses associated with generating print materials, even when they exclusively publish digital issues. This practice has been met with skepticism.
- *Impact on academic community*: The conventional framework of exorbitant expenses associated with non-open-access journal subscriptions places a considerable financial burden on the academic community, affecting institutions and individual researchers alike.
- *Limited support for authors*: While several open-access publishers offer reductions or exemptions for publishing fees to authors from underdeveloped nations or those facing financial difficulties, not all funding agencies provide such support. This can further exacerbate inequalities in publishing access.

- *Exclusion from funding*: Some funding agencies decline to provide financial support for additional expenses associated with open-access publication, such as APCs. This lack of coverage may hinder researchers' ability to publish their work in open-access journals.
- *The Diamond Open Access model*: The emergence of the Diamond Open Access model, which offers free and unrestricted access to research articles without financial barriers, has garnered attention. However, this model also faces questions about its sustainability and representation in scholarly databases.

In conclusion, the financial implications of scientific publishing have given rise to various criticisms, from concerns about transparency and incentives to questions about funding priorities and unequal access. As the publishing landscape continues to evolve, addressing these criticisms will be essential to ensure equitable access to research and maintain the integrity of scientific publishing.

IMPACT OF FEE CHOICES ON RESEARCH

When navigating the landscape of scientific publishing, the choices you make regarding fees can significantly influence the outcome and impact of your research. Understanding how these choices affect various aspects of your academic journey is crucial. In this section, we will delve into the key considerations related to the impact of fee choices on your research.

Balancing Quality and Cost-effectiveness

One of the primary considerations when dealing with publication fees is striking the right balance between quality and cost-effectiveness. Here are some points to ponder:

Quality of journals: While cost-effective options are appealing, it is vital to prioritize the quality and reputation of the journals you choose. Opting for reputable journals, even if they have higher fees, can enhance the visibility and credibility of your research.

Peer review and editing: Some journals with lower fees may cut corners in peer review and editing processes. Investing in journals that provide rigorous peer review and professional editing services can improve the overall quality of your published work.

Research funding: Consider the source of funding for your research. If you have research grants or institutional support, you may have more flexibility in selecting journals with higher fees that offer greater visibility and impact.

Ensuring Your Research Reaches the Right Audience

The ultimate goal of publishing your research is to share your findings with the relevant academic community and beyond. Fee choices can impact the dissemination of your work:

Target audience: Identify your target audience and choose journals that cater to that specific academic community. Publishing in journals aligned with your research area ensures that your work reaches those most interested in it.

Open access versus subscription: Decide whether open-access or subscription-based journals are more suitable for your goals. Open-access journals make your work freely accessible to a global audience, potentially increasing its impact, while subscription-based journals may limit access to subscribers.

Long-term Considerations for Your Academic Career

Your decisions regarding publication fees can have lasting effects on your academic career. Here is what to keep in mind:

Visibility and impact: Publishing in well-regarded journals, even if they have higher fees, can enhance the visibility and impact of your work. This can lead to more citations, collaborations, and career opportunities.

Career advancement: Consider the publication choices that align with your career goals. Some academic institutions and tenure committees value publications in certain journals or types of journals more than others. Research the expectations and criteria relevant to your career advancement.

Budgeting: Long-term budgeting is crucial. Assess your financial situation and allocate resources for publication fees as part of your research expenses. Strategic planning ensures you can continue to publish in journals that align with your academic goals.

RESOURCES FOR FEE INFORMATION

Accessing information about publication fees is essential for making informed decisions. Fortunately, numerous resources are available to assist researchers in navigating the fee structure of scientific publishing. Some valuable resources to consider are mentioned in the following text.

Online Databases and Directories

ThinkCheckSubmit.org: This online platform offers a comprehensive and systematic approach to assessing the quality of academic journals, including information on publication fees.

DOAJ: This provides a searchable repository of esteemed open-access journals and their fee structures, helping you identify suitable venues for your research.

COPE: This offers information on ethical publishing practices, which can indirectly influence fee transparency and quality.

Consulting with Mentors and Colleagues

Academic mentors: Seek guidance from experienced mentors in your field. They can provide insights into reputable journals and their fee structures, based on their own publishing experiences.

Colleagues: Discuss fee-related experiences with colleagues who have published in similar areas. Sharing information can help you make informed decisions.

Staying Up-to-date with Fee Trends

Scholarly publications: Regularly read scholarly articles, blogs, and publications that discuss trends and issues related to publication fees. Being aware of the evolving landscape can help you adapt your strategies.

Professional organizations: Join relevant academic and professional organizations in your field. Many of these organizations provide resources and updates on publishing practices, including fee-related matters.

By considering these factors and utilizing the available resources, you can make well-informed decisions regarding publication fees that align with your research goals and career aspirations. Balancing cost-effectiveness, audience reach, and long-term career considerations is essential for successful scientific publishing.[6]

CONCLUSION

- *Recap of key points*: In this chapter, we have explored the intricate landscape of publication fees and how they impact the world of scientific publishing. Let us recap the key points we have discussed:
  - *Types of fees*: We have distinguished between various publication fees, including APCs, submission fees, page charges, and color figure charges.
  - *Open access versus subscription*: We have examined the differences between open-access and subscription-based publishing models and how they relate to publication fees.
  - *Predatory journals*: We have highlighted the importance of identifying predatory journals and the risks associated with them, including excessive fees and poor quality.
  - *Ethical considerations*: We have emphasized the ethical aspects of fee structures, focusing on transparency, avoiding predatory publishers, and recognizing hidden or excessive fees.
  - *Impact on research*: We have explored how fee choices can affect research quality, audience reach, and long-term academic careers.
  - *Resources*: We have provided resources and strategies to help beginners navigate the fee structure effectively.

- *The evolving landscape of publication fees*: The landscape of publication fees is continually evolving. New publishing models, funding strategies, and technologies are reshaping how research is disseminated. As we move forward, here are some trends to keep in mind:
    - *Emergence of Diamond Open Access*: The Diamond Open Access model, which provides unrestricted access to research articles without author-facing fees, is gaining traction. Researchers are encouraged to explore this model's potential benefits and limitations.
    - *Greater fee transparency*: The academic community is pushing for greater transparency in fee structures. Publishers are increasingly expected to provide clear information about costs, waivers, and discounts.
    - *Innovations in peer review*: New peer review models, such as transparent peer review and post-publication peer review, are influencing how journals allocate their resources and, subsequently, their fee structures.
    - *Funding shifts*: Funding agencies are reconsidering their support for publication fees, potentially impacting researchers' choices and access to publishing venues.
- *Empowering beginners to make informed choices*: As beginners in the world of scientific publication, you have the tools and knowledge needed to make informed choices about publication fees. Here's how you can empower yourselves:
    - *Stay informed*: Regularly update yourselves about changes in the publishing landscape. Be aware of emerging trends, ethical considerations, and the evolving fee structures.
    - *Use resources*: Leverage the resources available to you. Explore online databases, directories, and the advice of mentors and colleagues to find suitable publication venues.
    - *Prioritize quality*: Always prioritize the quality of the journal over the cost. Investing in reputable journals can benefit your research and career in the long run.
    - *Budget wisely*: Plan your research budget carefully, allocating resources for publication fees when necessary. Consider the impact of your publication choices on your academic journey.
    - *Promote transparency*: Advocate for transparency in fee structures. Encourage publishers to provide clear information about fees, waivers, and the peer review process.

In your journey as scientific authors, you play a vital role in shaping the future of scholarly communication. By making informed choices about publication fees, you contribute to a more transparent, equitable, and quality-driven publishing ecosystem. May your research reach its full potential and impact, advancing knowledge and innovation across the globe. Happy publishing!

REFERENCES

1. Chan L, Cuplinskas D, Eisen M, Friend F, Genova Y, Guédon JG, et al. Budapest open access initiative. Read the Declaration. [online] Available from http://www.budapestopenaccessinitiative.org/read [Last accessed January, 2024].
2. Davis PM, Lewenstein BV, Simon DH, Booth JG, Connolly MJ. Open access publishing, article downloads, and citations: randomized controlled trial. BMJ. 2008;337:a568.
3. Gershman S. (2014). Profit and loss: The exploitative economics of academic publishing. [online] Available from https://footnote.co/the-exploitative-economics-of-academic-publishing [Last accessed January, 2024].
4. Elmore SA, Weston EH. Predatory Journals: What They Are and How to Avoid Them. Toxicol Pathol. 2020;48(4):607-10.
5. Panitch JM, Michalak S. (2005). The Serials Crisis: A White Paper for the UNC-Chapel Hill Scholarly Communication Convocation. January, 2005. [online] Available from https://ils.unc.edu/courses/2019_fall/inls700_001/Readings/Panitch2005-SerialsCrisis.htm [Last accessed January, 2024].
6. Björk BC, Solomon D. Pricing principles used by Scholarly Open Access Publishers. Learned Publ. 2012;25(3):132-7.
7. Wallace WA. Publish and be damned: the damage being created by predatory publishing. Bone Joint J. 2019;101-B(5):500-1.

4

SECTION

Communication with the Journal

CHAPTER 16

How to Compose a Cover Letter and What are the Documents to be Uploaded along with the Manuscript?

Saibal Das

INTRODUCTION

Composing a cover letter and preparing the necessary documents to accompany your manuscript submission to a journal or publisher is an essential part of the publication process. Here is a step-by-step guide on how to compose a cover letter and what documents to include.[1-3]

COVER LETTER

A cover letter is your introduction to the journal or publisher. It should be professional, concise, and convey essential information. Here is how to compose an effective cover letter.

Header

- Include your contact information at the top of the letter, including your full name, address, phone number, and email address.
- *Date*: Add the current date below your contact information.

Salutation

Address the letter to the editor in chief or the appropriate editor by name if possible. If you are unsure, a generic salutation like "Dear (Journal Name) Editorial Team" can be used.

Opening Paragraph

- Start with a brief introduction of yourself and your affiliations (e.g., your university or research institution).
- Mention the title of your manuscript and specify that you are submitting it for consideration for publication in their journal or with their publishing house.

Middle Paragraph(s)

- Provide a brief summary of your research and its significance. Explain why your work is a good fit for their journal or publishing platform.
- Mention any unique aspects of your study or findings.
- Highlight any potential conflicts of interest or special considerations they should be aware of.
- State that the manuscript is not under consideration for publication elsewhere.

Closing Paragraph

- Express your appreciation for their consideration.
- Include any specific requests, such as suggesting preferred reviewers or stating that you have attached additional documents.
- Offer your contact information and express your willingness to provide further information if needed.

Closing

- Use a formal closing like "Sincerely" or "Yours faithfully".
- Sign the letter with your handwritten signature if submitting a physical copy; otherwise, type your name.

DOCUMENTS TO BE UPLOADED WITH THE MANUSCRIPT

The exact requirements may vary depending on the journal or publisher, so it is essential to check their submission guidelines carefully. However, some common documents to include are described in the following text.[4,5]

Manuscript

The main document containing your research paper, written according to the journal's formatting and style guidelines.

Cover Letter

Attach the cover letter you have composed.

Title Page

A separate page with the manuscript title, authors' names, affiliations, corresponding author's contact information, and any disclaimers or additional information required by the journal.

Abstract

A brief summary of your research, usually around 150–250 words.

Figures and Tables

Include any figures, graphs, tables, and captions as separate files, following the journal's formatting instructions.

References

List all the references cited in your manuscript in the appropriate citation style.

Supplementary Material

If applicable, include any supplementary materials (e.g., additional data, code, or appendices) as separate files.

Conflict of Interest Statement

If applicable, provide a statement regarding any conflicts of interest among the authors.

Ethical Statements

Include any required ethical statements, such as informed consent or ethical approval, as specified by the journal.

Always double-check the submission guidelines provided by the journal or publisher, as specific requirements may vary. Ensure that all documents are in the requested format and follow any additional instructions provided. This will increase your chances of a smooth and successful manuscript submission process.

FURTHER READINGS

1. Liumbruno GM, Velati C, Pasqualetti P, Franchini M. How to write a scientific manuscript for publication. Blood Transfus. 2013;11(2):217-26.
2. Gemayel R. How to write a scientific paper. FEBS J. 2016;283(21):3882-5.
3. Su'a B, MacFater WS, Hill AG. How to write a paper: revising your manuscript. ANZ J Surg. 2017;87(3):195-7.
4. Tomaska L. Teaching how to prepare a manuscript by means of rewriting published scientific papers. Genetics. 2007;175(1):17-20.
5. Kern MJ, Bonneau HN. Approach to manuscript preparation and submission: how to get your paper accepted. Catheter Cardiovasc Interv. 2003;58(3):391-6.

CHAPTER 17

How to Respond to Reviewer Queries?

Saibal Das

INTRODUCTION

Responding to reviewer queries or comments is a crucial part of the peer review process when you have submitted a manuscript to a journal. Reviewers provide feedback and raise questions to help improve the quality and clarity of your research paper. Here is a step-by-step guide on how to effectively respond to reviewer queries:

1. *Read the reviews carefully*: Take the time to thoroughly read through the reviewers' comments and suggestions. Ensure you understand each point they have raised.
2. *Stay professional and positive*: Approach the responses with professionalism and a positive attitude. Remember that reviewers are providing valuable input to help improve your work.
3. *Organize your responses*: Create a document or spreadsheet to organize your responses to each comment or query. List each reviewer's comment/question and your response alongside it.
4. *Acknowledge and thank the reviewers*: Begin your response by acknowledging the reviewers' feedback and expressing gratitude for their time and effort in reviewing your manuscript.
5. *Be specific and detailed*: Address each comment or query individually and in detail. Provide specific responses that demonstrate how you have addressed the reviewer's concerns or suggestions.
6. *Use a clear structure*: Structure your responses logically, following the same order as the reviewers' comments or numbering them for reference. This makes it easier for the reviewers to follow your responses.
7. *Provide evidence and explanations*: Backup your responses with evidence from your research, additional data, or references to relevant literature. Explain the rationale behind your decisions.

8. *Be transparent*: If you made changes to the manuscript in response to a reviewer's comment, clearly state what changes were made and where they can find these changes in the revised manuscript.
9. *Address all comments*: Ensure that you address every comment or query raised by the reviewers. If you disagree with a suggestion, explain your reasoning politely.
10. *Maintain a professional tone*: Maintain a respectful and professional tone in your responses, even if you disagree with a reviewer's feedback. Avoid getting defensive.
11. *Seek clarification (if needed)*: If you are uncertain about a reviewer's comment or need clarification, do not hesitate to ask the editor for clarification or for the reviewer's contact information to seek clarification directly (if the journal allows this).
12. *Proofread your responses*: Carefully proofread your responses for grammar, spelling, and clarity. Ensure your responses are well written and error-free.
13. *Meet deadlines*: Submit your responses within the specified time frame. If you need more time, communicate this to the editor promptly.
14. *Follow the journal's guidelines*: Adhere to any specific formatting or submission guidelines provided by the journal for your response letter.
15. *Revise your manuscript*: Make the necessary revisions to your manuscript based on your responses to the reviewers' comments. Ensure that these changes improve the quality and clarity of your paper.
16. *Reiterate your gratitude*: Close your response letter by thanking the reviewers and the editor for their time and feedback.

Once you have prepared your responses, submit them along with the revised manuscript to the journal through the submission system. Be prepared for further rounds of review if the reviewers have additional concerns or questions. Responding to reviewer queries effectively is an iterative process that can ultimately lead to the acceptance of your manuscript for publication.

5 SECTION

Publication Ethics

CHAPTER 18

Plagiarism and Copyright Issues

Chiranjib Bagchi

INTRODUCTION

To excel in the domain of research and education, skill of writing is an essential component. In fact, this skill should be honed from the years of studentship. But in present days, we are attracted to copy and share the interesting articles or publications in one click of mouse, which has become very easy with the availability of internet and modern technological gadgets. This practice is often reflected in the writing of a manuscript, by indulging into the "copy and paste menace." As per one large study (McCabe's, 2003) done in the United States and Canada, it is revealed that the percentage of students using "cut and paste internet sources" had increased from 13 to 41 since academic year 1999–2000 to 2001–2002, respectively.[1] Many times, the authors appear unaware of the intellectual property right (IPR) issues and get astonished upon being charged with plagiarism and copyright infringement clause.[2] Now, educationists agree that both teachers and the students should be aware of the IPR issues, irrespective of their scope of work in either arts or science or creative or scholarly works. For a researcher and academician, it is always "*better late than never*" to get familiarized with these concepts and learn the basics of IPR.

The word "plagiarism" is derived from the lattin word "plundering." It means "*Taking materials (artistic or academic work) from others for one's own purposes*" (Oxford language). Plagiarism has been defined in many ways: As per Oxford dictionary, it is defined as "*Take and use the thoughts, writings, inventions of another person as one's own, pass off the thoughts, etc. of another person as one's own.*" As per Merriam-Webster.com, plagiarism is defined as "*Using another person's words or ideas without giving credit to that person.*"

Besides this concept, plagiarism should be remembered to take several forms.

PLAGIARISM INFOGRAPHIC

Ten common types of plagiarism infographic are:[3,4]

1. *Clone (direct)*: Copying word-to-word, keeping same as the original, without citing the source
2. *Remix (potluck)*: When paraphrasing is done using the contents from different sources ending up to a write-up that fits together impeccably
3. *404 error*: Using citations from sources that do not exist—the name is adopted from the error message received on searching some invalid sources online.
4. *Retweet*: When most of the original text wording and sentence is copied.
5. *Hybrid*: When a document is created with a well-resourced content, utilizing many sources without citing all the texts, landing up attributing fewer sources than actually used.
6. *Ctrl-C*: In majority of the documents, the plagiarized text appears almost similar to the original text with a few changes, more or less same to cloning, except minimal changes are made in the text.
7. *Find-replace (mosaic)*: Interestingly, here the synonyms are used to replace the key words and phrases of the original text.
8. *Recycle*: It is a modest form of plagiarism where the author presents a previously produced content without providing the citation properly. The other name of this is self-plagiarism.
9. *Mashup*: Here, the content is prepared using different sources but presented without citing those sources appropriately.
10. *Aggregator*: Here, the author attributes sources with proper citations, but the whole content is mostly composed of contents from other sources without any original content.

PLAGIARISM—FEW EXAMPLES[5]

- Failure to acknowledge the author or a person while copying or quoting him or her from the online sources, a published article, or an interview
- Copying a substantial part of one's write-up or work without citing the article or source
- Copying or buying a paper and sharing it as one's own
- Falsely creating a citation that does not exist
- Paraphrasing someone else's thoughts or ideas without giving due credit or citing
- Depending much on original author's language or syntax while paraphrasing the content

Now, the next question is how plagiarism differs from copyright infringement. Basically, the difference lies in the conceptual level. An idea or thought cannot be copyrighted under the law. Raw data do not get protection under copyright, instead data are protected when they are organized in database. Thus, copying an idea, thought, or data is not copyright infringement but can be a case of plagiarism. Interestingly in India, currently, there is no law to punish plagiarism. As an example, making and selling of a pirated or copied book is not considered as plagiarism, it is copyright infringement. But if the copied book is sold also in the name of the copier without recognizing the original author, it turns out to be both copyright infringement and plagiarism.

Similarly, suppose, two authors jointly write an article and publish in a journal after surrendering the copyright to the publisher; subsequently, one author writes and publishes an article in another journal where there is overlapping of some contents from the previous article, but no permission from the previous publisher is taken nor the coauthor is acknowledged—here, misappropriation of joint authorship has happened and it is a clear case of copyright infringement.[6] So, while signing the assignment form, the terms and conditions of the authorship and publication policy of the journal should be reviewed carefully by the authors before surrendering the copyright of the article to the publisher.

COPYRIGHT INFRINGEMENT VIS-À-VIS PLAGIARISM[5,7]

Copyright infringement encompasses unauthorized or unlicensed copying of a copyrighted work (Tech Law Journal).

Plagiarism is copying others' work or ideas without giving him or her due credit and presenting the idea or thought as one's own.

Plagiarism is considered as ethical violation or ethical malpractice, but infringement bears a legal connotation too.

Plagiarism is not illegal; it is a violation of academic norms, whereas copyright violation or infringement is very common in academia but illegal.

As in traditional academic publishing, copyright transfer agreement (CTA) has been a common practice; the copyright holder and author are not always the same. Thus, plagiarism is an "act of offense" against the author and copyright infringement is conducted against the copyright holder.

Plagiarism happens when anybody is copying others' work or ideas—common in academic setting (schools or colleges), professional (publication, job-related work), or creative settings. Here, mainly ethical issues are involved, a breach of intellectual honesty becomes apparent, and academic and or disciplinary actions such as warnings may be undertaken.

Copyright infringement activity violates the rights under possession by the creators (or copyright holders) over certain types of work ensured by the copyright and intellectual property laws. It involves a legal consideration and a commercial interest may underlie.

Copied ideas are plagiarism, whereas copying a fixed specific expression (whole sequence of words or image) is copyright violation.

Plagiarism can be avoided by judiciously sharing the intellectual credit and copyright infringement can be avoided without disturbing the ways how the revenue is generated by an individual or company.

Problem situations: In plagiarism, copying the work or ideas of others without attribution, poorly paraphrasing the work of others, and substantial amount or intentional copying can create problems. In copyright infringement, problem may arise when copyrighted work is used beyond the permissible limit and without any permission of the copyright holder. Moreover, problem may also arise either when an unauthorized copying or distribution of a copyrighted work is contemplated.

For examples, plagiarism—if a large portion or word-to-word is copied from another work; *copyright infringement*—copying a computer program software without the copyright holder's permission and sharing it to others.

Consequences: Plagiarism—disciplinary action—loss of a job. Copyright infringement—takedown notice and civil lawsuit, as well criminal action may be for intentional circumstances where profiteering is involved.

Minimizing the risk: Plagiarism—utilizing acceptable portion of one's work or ideas in support of creating a new one. Paraphrasing or summarizing someone's ideas or work is recommended. Properly citing the sources using the standard style is recommended. Copyright infringement—prior evaluation for using that work under the clause of exception is encouraged and if not, then obtaining permission and providing attribution while using it is highly recommended.

Public domain works: Public domain works do not hold copyright, but appropriate attribution provides recognition to the creator and intellectual property is respected.

WAYS TO AVOID PLAGIARISM

To avoid accusations of plagiarism, credit is to be given whenever anyone uses. The ways to avoid plagiarism are:[5]

- Someone's idea, opinion, or theory
- Any information, facts, statistical data, graphical presentations, or images that are not common knowledge
- Quotations of another person's actual spoken or written words
- Paraphrase of another person's spoken or written words

FEW MORE TIPS

- Source of information in the publications/works should be traced (author, article title, journal name, book publisher, and publication date).
- The uniform resource locator (URL) where the information is found should be recorded along with the date of accessing the website.
- All the abovementioned information should be properly preserved until the paper is finalized.

- The sources should be cited properly, following the correct referencing style (Vancouver or Harvard or others).

With the availability of good software, copyright infringement and plagiarism can be easily detected. The style guide is to be followed meticulously. There should be a clear marking of the direct quotes; additionally, those are to be cited properly. But paraphrasing the cited information in the direct quotes can also be done. In any case, the information must be cited.

Copyright infringement in India: "As per the Copyright Act, 1957, the use of a copyrighted work without the permission of the owner results in copyright infringement." Copying the work of one author intentionally or unintentionally by another one without giving any credit is copyright infringement. Primary and secondary infringements are the two categories. When actual copying occurs, it is considered as primary infringement, whereas unauthorized dealings such as selling or importing a pirated book constitutes secondary infringement. The infringer becomes aware in case of secondary infringement, whereas in case of primary infringement, he or she may remain unaware.

ELEMENTS FOR COPYRIGHT INFRINGEMENT[8]

- The author of the copyrighted work is the original creator.
- Copyright infringement occurs when the work is copied from the original one.

INSTANCES WHERE COPYRIGHT INFRINGEMENT OCCURS

Copyright Infringement Act of India (1957) states that violation of copyright occurs when:[9]

- Copyrighted works are sold or hired (online piracy) without permission.
- Copies are distributed for trading purpose or vested interest.
- Copyrighted work is reproduced in a public place.
- Pirated copies are imported to India from outside.
- Public exhibition of the copyrighted work
- Reproduction of a drama, literature, or artistic work

PLAGIARISM AND COPYRIGHT INFRINGEMENT: INDIAN LAWS AND REGULATIONS[8,9]

Indian Copyright Act, 1957, provides protection of the "literary works" and the courts have repeatedly clarified over the years that research theses and dissertations by the students, research reports, laboratory notebooks in research, questionnaire collecting statistical information, etc., come under the purview of this law. The punishments for copyright infringement under the act are not only restrictive measure of injunction but also amount to damages, fine, or imprisonment **(Fig. 1)**.

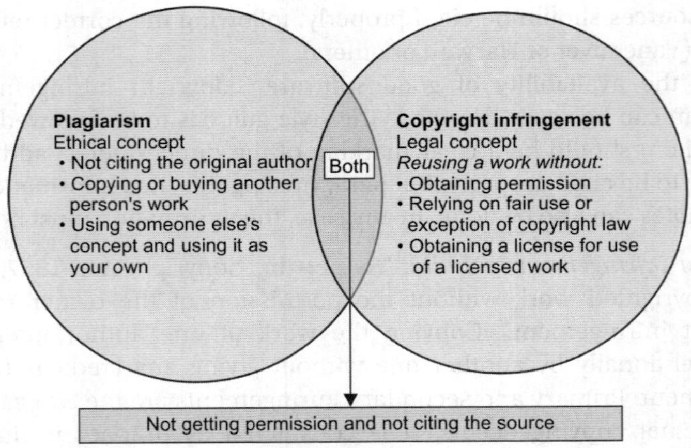

FIG. 1: Plagiarism and copyright infringement.

If anyone quotes a limited portion of others' work with due credit, it is acceptable. If copied substantially without any acknowledgement or due credit, the offender can be taken to the court. This may lead to injunctions to prevent copyright infringement. In India, copyright act is enacted under section 57 and is currently in force.

If the offender has earned from publication of the work, the original author can recover the damages if the case has definite merit. But if breaching the copyright is proved to be unintentional, the case might get dismissed **(Flowchart 1)**.

CONCLUSION

Intentional plagiarism and copyright infringement are in occurrence, but there are ways to deal with them appropriately. However in many instances, these are unintentional and happening due to lack of knowledge and awareness of students and faculties regarding these issues. The students can be allowed to take up projects on their interest areas so that they can diligently search for the references and originally contribute in writing; thus, they can be well motivated to take up their work seriously with freedom.

According to Hill (2017), "*The responsibility to ensure an ethical approach to academia must be shared. Students have a role to play but institutions cannot assume their levels of knowledge or understanding. Punishing the student without providing learning opportunities or access to information is neither efficient nor pedagogically sound.*"

The institution and the authorities can provide the sources and tools to discover new methods and technologies to check the scripts. They should provide a student's handbook focusing on the ways of restricting plagiarism, which may attract students.

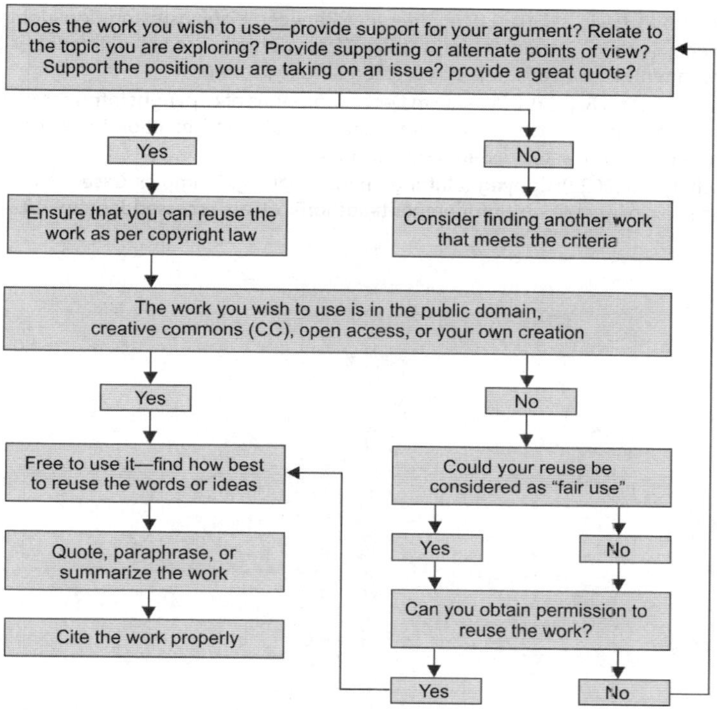

FLOWCHART 1: How to reuse any document.
Source: Adapted from Myers CS (2018).[3]

The students and faculties should seek assistance from the librarians to learn more about plagiarism and copyright infringement issues and the ways to avoid the same and how to reuse others' works with ethical and legal compliance.

REFERENCES

1. Ahmad T, Ghosh I. (2011). Plagiarism and Copyright Infringement. [online] Available from https://ssrn.com/abstract=1839353 [Last accessed January, 2024].
2. Crews KD. (Ed). Copyright Law for Librarians and Educators: Creative Strategies and Practical Solutions. USA: ALA Editions; 2020. pp. 320.
3. Myers CS (Ed). Plagiarism and Copyright: Best Practices for Classroom Education. UK: Routledge, Taylor & Francis Group; 2018. pp. 91-9.
4. Top Ten Types of Plagiarism Infographic. [online] Available from http://blog.plagiarismsearch.com/top-ten-most-popular-types-of-plagiarism [Last accessed January, 2024].
5. University of Illinois Chicago. (2023). Avoiding Plagiarism: Dissertation/Thesis FAQ re: Copyright [online] Available from https://researchguides.uic.edu/c.php?g=252209&p=1682802 [Last accessed, January 2024].
6. Saha R. Plagiarism, Research Publications and Law. Curr Sci. 2017;112(12):2375-8.

7. Arnold M, Levin S. (2021). The Difference Between Plagiarism and Copyright Infringement. [online] Available from https://copyrightalliance.org/differences-copyright-infringement-plagiarism/ [Last accessed January, 2024].
8. Parthasarathi R. (2019). Plagiarism Detection: Issues of copyright infringement. [online] Available from https://ceerapub.nls.ac.in/plagiarism-detection-issues-of-copyright-infringement/ [Last accessed January, 2024].
9. Acharya M (2022). Copyright Infringement: Meaning, Examples, Cases in India. https://cleartax.in/s/copyright-infringement#authorBio. [Last accessed January, 2024].

CHAPTER 19

Authorship

Nandini Chatterjee

INTRODUCTION

A publication is accompanied by the names of its authors on the byline, i.e., the line below the title. Authorship gives credit; however, it also entails accountability for published work.

It is important to have a clear conception about the various aspects of authorship while embarking on the journey of scientific publication as there are significant academic, social, and at times, financial implications.

Multiple authorship is the order of the day as any research nowadays is accomplished by the conjoint efforts of many individuals, through multidisciplinary teams, acquiring information from various sources.

There is also an academic hierarchy in research projects where students function under the guidance of their mentors. It becomes important to give credit to each and every person involved.

Single authorship was in vogue till the 1920s, where individual discoveries or observations were reported; however, as we know, there are several steps of manuscript preparation and documentation of work. It is imperative to involve multiple persons in the analysis and interpretation of data followed by drafting, revision, and final approval before publication.

WHO IS AN AUTHOR?

The International Committee of Medical Journal Editors (ICMJE) has developed four definite criteria for authorship, all of which need to be satisfied for an individual to be designated as author. The ICMJE recommends that authorship be based on the following four criteria:

1. Substantial contributions to the conception or design of the work or the acquisition, analysis, or interpretation of data for the work
2. Drafting the work or revising it critically for important intellectual content

3. Final approval of the version to be published
4. Agreement to be accountable for all aspects of the work in ensuring that questions related to the accuracy or integrity of any part of the work are appropriately investigated and resolved.[1,2]

WHAT ARE THE RESPONSIBILITIES OF AN AUTHOR?

It is mandatory that the group of authors should be able to take public responsibility for the accuracy and integrity of the study.

It is the collective duty of the authors to ensure that the names in the byline of the article satisfy all four criteria; it is to be remembered that journal editors are not supposed to determine authorship eligibility or to arbitrate authorship conflicts.

If there is ambiguity or disagreement about authorship, it is the responsibility of where the study was undertaken to investigate and settle the issues.

Some journals have a specific contributorship policy and publish separately the individual contributions of each author during the study and manuscript preparation. This ensures that there is no ambiguity about their inclusion and order of placement.[3]

WHO IS NOT AN AUTHOR?

The ICMJE criteria also help to distinguish authors from other contributors who are designated as nonauthor contributors.

We should keep in mind that there are certain actions, such as technical help, administrative assistance, proofreading, and fund acquisition, which are not considered criteria for authorship. These individuals need to be acknowledged at the end of the article.

At times, journals may ask for written permissions to be taken from all acknowledged individuals whose names will be uploaded by the corresponding author. This is to avoid controversy, as acknowledgement implies endorsement of the findings of the study.

HOW TO DECIDE THE ORDER OF AUTHORSHIP?

The order in which authors are listed is a collective decision by the authors through a consensus by mutual discussion. The criteria for deciding the order of authors are variable and need consent within the author group.

The quality and quantity of effort put into the research and manuscript preparation is to be taken into account and this decision should be taken even before the work has actually begun by allotment of specific responsibilities. Collective discussion is very important in avoiding dissent and bitterness. The National Medical Commission (NMC) currently gives credit to the first, second, and third authors along with the corresponding author in the promotional considerations of individuals in service.

WHAT IS THE JOB OF THE CORRESPONDING AUTHOR?

Of all the authors, the corresponding author plays a vital role in communicating with the journal, responding to queries about the publication during the review process and also afterward should there be any need for additional data.

All documents, such as the details of authors, ethics committee approval, clinical trial registration, and relevant disclosures, also need to be furnished by the corresponding author.

The corresponding author has immense responsibility to respond to reviewer queries and comments. The responses should address each query systematically with a stipulated time frame. He or she should furnish all data or additional information as per request of the journal even after publication.

The corresponding author must also disclose, at submission, whether any information or figure in the manuscript has been previously published elsewhere. It is mandatory to provide written permission from authors of the prior work and/or publishers.

After acceptance, the corresponding author is responsible for the accuracy of all content in the proof, including the names of coauthors, addresses, and affiliations. Although the corresponding author has primary responsibility for correspondence with the journal, the ICMJE recommends that editors send copies of all correspondence to all listed authors.[1,2]

HOW TO DESIGNATE THE CORRESPONDING AUTHOR?

The authors should authorize the corresponding author to reply to all communications from the journal or the reviewers on their behalf. All the details, namely name of the corresponding author, email address, phone number, and postal address are to be furnished.

Many journals have an authorization form where all authors acknowledge that they have read the criteria for authorship and fulfill the four criteria of authorship and they authorize the corresponding author for necessary changes and communications with the journal.

It is desirable to provide the Open Researcher and Contributor Identifier (ORCID) of the corresponding authors of published papers as also that of the coauthors. This enhances the validity and credibility of the paper.

HOW TO CARRY OUT ANY CHANGE IN AUTHORSHIP?

If any alteration to the order of the authors or the removal or addition of authors after submission is contemplated, consent from all coauthors is required.

It is to be communicated with the journal by the corresponding author. Journal editors may ask for a signed declaration for the requested change from all the authors and also from the author(s) who are to be removed or added.

However, it is to be remembered that changes of authorship are usually not permitted after acceptance of a manuscript.

WHAT IS CONSORTIA AUTHORSHIP?

A consortium is a group of authors listed together as a collective entity. All authors within a consortium need to be mentioned individually at the bottom of the paper.

WHO IS A GUEST AUTHOR?

It is a common occurrence in reality that the names on the byline do not reflect the strict recommendations mentioned earlier. Many times, the guest authors and gift authors find pride of place in the authorship lineup.

The guest authors are usually influential people whose inclusion in the byline may be a way to increase the credibility of the publication.

Gift authors are people who feature in the list due to some personal rapport and senior authors might want to reward someone who has helped them in the past or gratify coworkers to maintain cordial relations with them. At times, junior authors may put a senior colleague's name with the hope of favorable consequences regarding review and publication.[4]

WHO IS A GHOST AUTHOR?

Ghost authors are those who contribute to the research, data analysis, and/or manuscript preparation but are not credited as authors of the article. This may at times be a student or junior scientist or a medical writer employed by some company. This is a breach in the code of publication ethics but rampant nonetheless.

WHAT IS THE STATUS OF ARTIFICIAL INTELLIGENCE IN AUTHORSHIP?

Nowadays, artificial intelligence (AI)-assisted technologies [such as large language models (LLMs), chatbots, or image creators] are often utilized in the preparation of manuscripts. It is ethical to mention in both the cover letter and the submitted work how AI had been used.

As of now, AI and AI-assisted technologies cannot be mentioned as author or coauthor. The responsibility to vouch for the authenticity of the work rests on the humans who are answerable to any queries regarding the submitted manuscript.

Authors should ensure there is no plagiarism in the text and images produced by the AI and full citations are to be provided for all materials included.

WHAT ARE THE MOTIVATIONS OF AUTHORS BEHIND PUBLICATIONS?

Communication to the scientific world about one's own research work is the most important; but at times, it may be a pressure to increase chances of getting research grants, promotions in academic career, or tenure positions.

All this leads to a large number of authors in publications, a condition called hyperauthorship.

However, it should be kept in mind that though an authorship may bring reputation to a person, it also entails responsibilities of defending the intellectual content of the manuscript, concede any error publicly, and in case of fraud, state publicly its extent and nature and why it occurred.

ARE THERE ETHICAL ISSUES REGARDING AUTHORSHIP?

The Committee on Publication Ethics (COPE) has guidelines and advisories for authors, as well as journal editors for guidance regarding various responsibilities of authors. Awareness about the criteria and responsibility of authorship is becoming very essential nowadays. The author should know, understand, and adhere to recommendations laid down by ICMJE.

Flowcharts for detecting authorship problems, should disputes arise, are also readily available. All information about recommendations and guidelines of the ICMJE and COPE are available on the public domain and may be downloaded for personal upgradation and knowledge before one embarks on the next manuscript preparation.

REFERENCES

1. ICMJE. (2013). The new ICMJE recommendations. [online] Available from http://www.icmje.org/news-and-editorials/new_rec_aug2013.html [Last accessed January, 2024].
2. ICMJE. (2016). Recommendations for the conduct, reporting, editing, and publication of scholarly work in medical journals. [online] Available from http://www.icmje.org/index.html [Last accessed January, 2024].
3. Jones AH. Can authorship policies help prevent scientific misconduct? What role for scientific societies? Sci Eng Ethics. 2003;9:243-56.
4. Helgesson G, Eriksson S. Responsibility for scientific misconduct in collaborative papers. Med Health Care Philos. 2018;21(3):423-30.

CHAPTER 20

Disclosures, Conflict of Interest, Scientific Misconduct, and Retraction in Scientific Writing

Shreyashi Dasgupta, Santanu K Tripathi, Shambo Samrat Samajdar

INTRODUCTION

Scientific writing plays a crucial role in the advancement of knowledge and the dissemination of information. Whether it is a research paper, a thesis, a scientific article, or a laboratory report, the way scientists communicate their findings impacts the understanding and trust of the broader scientific community and the public. Disclosures in scientific writing are therefore vital for maintaining honesty, integrity, and transparency in research.

SCIENTIFIC RESEARCH AND ITS IMPACT

Scientific research is the engine that drives progress in fields ranging from medicine and technology to environmental science and social sciences. It involves formulating hypotheses, conducting experiments, and analyzing data to uncover new information and expand our collective knowledge. But, for this system to work effectively, it relies heavily on the honesty and transparency of researchers.

ROLE OF DISCLOSURES

Disclosures, in the context of scientific writing, refer to the information provided by researchers about their methodologies, funding sources, potential conflicts of interest, and any limitations or shortcomings in their work. These disclosures serve several important functions:

- *Honesty and integrity*: The cornerstone of scientific research is the pursuit of truth. When researchers disclose their methods, results, and potential conflicts, they demonstrate their commitment to honesty and integrity. This not only upholds the credibility of the individual researcher but also the entire scientific community.

- *Transparency*: Transparency is essential for building trust. By disclosing their research methods and potential sources of bias or error, scientists allow other researchers to critically evaluate their work. This transparency encourages healthy skepticism, peer review, and the replication of studies, which are all fundamental to the scientific method.
- *Ethical considerations*: Disclosures are a way to address ethical concerns in research. For example, if a study involving human subjects did not obtain informed consent, disclosing this can help identify ethical breaches. Furthermore, researchers must disclose any potential conflicts of interest that might compromise the objectivity of their work.
- *Accountability*: Researchers are accountable not only to their peers but also to the general public and policymakers who may use their findings to make decisions. Disclosures help ensure that researchers are answerable for the quality of their work and the potential consequences of their findings.

TYPES OF DISCLOSURES

There are several key types of disclosures that researchers should include in their scientific writing:[1,2]

- *Methodological disclosures*: Researchers must provide detailed descriptions of the methods and techniques they used in their studies. This includes the materials, procedures, and statistical analyses employed. A lack of clarity in this area can make it difficult for others to reproduce the study and evaluate its validity.
- *Funding sources*: Researchers should disclose the sources of funding for their projects. External funding can introduce potential biases, and transparency in this regard is critical to maintaining trust in the research.
- *Conflicts of interest*: It is essential for researchers to acknowledge any personal, financial, commercial, political or professional interests that may influence the outcome of their work. Research funding, employment, stock or shareholding, monetary support for travel or lectures may all constitute potential areas of conflict of interest. Failure to disclose conflicts of interest can undermine the credibility of the research.
- *Limitations and shortcomings*: No study is perfect, and researchers should openly discuss the limitations and shortcomings of their work. This can include sample size, data collection issues, or the potential for bias. Acknowledging these limitations helps other researchers and readers interpret the results accurately.
- *Ethical considerations*: If a study involved human or animal subjects, it is crucial to disclose adherence to ethical standards and guidelines. This includes obtaining informed consent in clinical studies and following established ethical review processes.
- *Data sharing and availability*:[3] In recent years, the scientific community has increasingly recognized the importance of data sharing. Researchers

are encouraged to make their data available for other scientists to scrutinize, verify, and build upon. Disclosures related to data sharing, or the lack thereof, can significantly impact the credibility of a study.

When data is not shared, it becomes challenging for others to independently assess the research's validity. Data availability enhances transparency and allows for the potential discovery of errors or fraud. Research articles should specify whether the data is accessible, and if so, where it can be found.

IMPORTANCE OF METHODOLOGICAL DISCLOSURES

Methodological disclosures are at the heart of scientific writing. The methodology section of a research paper or article provides a roadmap for how the study was conducted. This section is critical because it allows other researchers to understand, evaluate, and potentially replicate the study. The importance of detailed methodological disclosures cannot be overstated.

For example: A medical researcher publishes a study claiming that a new drug is highly effective at treating a particular disease. Without a clear and thorough methodology section, other scientists cannot replicate the experiment to verify the results. Furthermore, if the methodology is flawed or biased in some way, it may lead to erroneous conclusions that could have serious implications for patient care.

In addition to enabling replication, methodological disclosures also allow for a critical evaluation of the study. Other researchers can assess whether the methods used were appropriate and whether the data collection and analysis were conducted rigorously. This scrutiny is a fundamental aspect of the peer review process, which is essential for maintaining the quality and integrity of scientific research. Disclosure of methodology is especially important in case of negative results, where it adds value to such results by enabling critical review of the research process.[4]

SIGNIFICANCE OF DISCLOSURES

Disclosures serve as the building blocks of trust in scientific literature. When researchers provide accurate and comprehensive disclosures, they enable readers to critically evaluate the research, understand potential sources of bias, and assess the reliability of the findings. This transparency fosters accountability, ethical conduct, and the responsible dissemination of knowledge.

Transparency Enhances Accountability

Accountability is a cornerstone of scientific research. It ensures that researchers are held responsible for their actions and that the public can trust the outcomes of their work. Disclosures play a pivotal role in this process by revealing potential conflicts of interest, funding sources, and ethical considerations.

When researchers are transparent about their funding sources, it becomes easier to track the origins of financial support and identify any undue influence that may have affected the research. This accountability helps prevent the misdirection of research agendas toward profit-driven or biased goals.

Furthermore, disclosing conflicts of interest ensures that researchers remain impartial and objective in their work. This transparency allows the scientific community and the public to assess the potential influence of personal or professional interests on the research's validity. In doing so, it guards against ethical lapses and maintains the integrity of scientific investigations.

Transparency Promotes Ethical Conduct

Ethical conduct is a nonnegotiable aspect of scientific research. Disclosures related to informed consent, ethical review board approvals, and adherence to ethical guidelines are essential to ensure that research is conducted with the utmost integrity and respect for the rights and well-being of participants.

For instance, when researchers provide information about obtaining informed consent from human subjects, they demonstrate their commitment to respecting the autonomy and rights of those involved in the study. This transparency reassures readers that the research was conducted ethically and in compliance with established standards.

In cases involving animal research, ethical disclosures are equally important. They convey the researchers' adherence to humane practices and ethical guidelines, emphasizing the welfare of animals involved in the study.

Transparency Supports the Responsible Dissemination of Knowledge

Scientific knowledge has the power to shape public policies, drive technological advancements, and influence decision-making at various levels. Therefore, the responsible dissemination of knowledge is vital to ensure that the public and policymakers can rely on accurate and unbiased information.

Disclosures in scientific writing contribute to the responsible dissemination of knowledge by allowing readers to make informed judgments about the research. This is particularly crucial in areas where public health and safety are at stake. For example, the pharmaceutical industry's disclosure of clinical trial results, both positive and negative, is essential for healthcare professionals and regulators to make informed decisions about drug safety and efficacy.

Additionally, when data is made available for others to review and analyze, it encourages collaboration and strengthens the foundation of scientific knowledge. Reproducibility and the validation of research findings become feasible, ultimately enhancing the robustness of scientific understanding.

Challenges and Concerns[5,6]

While the importance of disclosures in scientific writing is clear, there are challenges and concerns associated with their implementation.

- *Incomplete or inaccurate disclosures*: One of the primary concerns is the possibility of incomplete or inaccurate disclosures. Some researchers may be tempted to conceal conflicts of interest, funding sources, or ethical lapses. This can lead to a lack of trust in scientific literature and a potential misallocation of resources, both of which are detrimental to the scientific community and society at large. When disclosures are lacking or inadequate, it can lead to a variety of problems, both within the scientific community and in the broader public perception of science.
- *Reproducibility crisis*: In recent years, there has been growing concern about the reproducibility of scientific studies. Inadequate methodological disclosures make it challenging for other researchers to replicate experiments, which can erode confidence in the reliability of scientific findings.
- *Misinterpretation*: Without clear methodological disclosures, there is a risk that the results of a study may be misinterpreted or misapplied. This can have serious consequences, particularly in fields like medicine, where incorrect information can harm patients.
- *Distrust in science*: Inadequate disclosures can contribute to a perception that scientific research is not transparent or trustworthy. This can lead to a decline in public trust in the scientific community and reluctance to accept scientific consensus on important issues like climate change or vaccines.
- *Ethical concerns*: Failure to disclose conflicts of interest or ethical breaches can result in not only scientific but also legal and ethical consequences for researchers. It can damage reputations and, in some cases, lead to investigations and sanctions.
- *Wastage of resources*: Incomplete disclosures can waste valuable time and resources. Researchers may attempt to build upon a study with inadequate disclosures, only to discover that it cannot be replicated or that the findings are not as claimed.
- *Data sharing hurdles*: Data sharing, while crucial for transparency and accountability, can be challenging to implement in practice. Researchers may face obstacles related to data privacy, intellectual property rights, and proprietary interests. Balancing the need for data sharing with these concerns is an ongoing debate in the scientific community.
- *Peer review limitations*: Peer review is a crucial quality control mechanism in scientific publishing. However, it may not always catch incomplete or inaccurate disclosures, especially if the reviewers themselves are unaware of potential conflicts or bias. Researchers, editors, and reviewers all play a role in ensuring thorough disclosures.

- *Legal and ethical dilemmas*: Researchers often grapple with legal and ethical dilemmas related to disclosures. While transparency is essential, it may raise concerns about intellectual property protection, patent applications, or contractual obligations with funding sources. Striking the right balance between transparency and these considerations is a complex task.
- *Reader interpretation*: Readers may vary in their ability to interpret and assess disclosures. Some may lack the expertise to fully understand the implications of certain disclosures, such as the influence of specific funding sources or conflicts of interest. Improving scientific communication and education can help address this challenge.

BEST PRACTICES FOR DISCLOSURES

To address these challenges and concerns, the scientific community has developed several best practices for disclosures in scientific writing:[7-9]

- *Clear and comprehensive reporting*: Researchers should provide clear, comprehensive, and easily accessible disclosures. Journal publishers and academic institutions can play a role in setting guidelines and standards for the information that must be disclosed in research articles.
- *Editorial oversight*: Journal editors and publishers have a responsibility to ensure that disclosures are complete and accurate. This includes the verification of funding sources, conflicts of interest, and ethical considerations. Journals can adopt policies that encourage adherence to these standards.
- *Peer review*: Peer reviewers should be trained to identify potential conflicts of interest and critically assess the completeness of disclosures. Their feedback can play a vital role in improving the transparency and quality of scientific publications.
- *Data sharing platforms*: Creating user-friendly data sharing platforms can facilitate the responsible sharing of research data. These platforms should address privacy concerns, intellectual property issues, and provide guidelines for data citation and usage.
- *Education and training*: Research institutions and organizations should prioritize education and training on ethical conduct, data sharing, and the importance of disclosures. This will help researchers navigate the complex landscape of scientific publishing while upholding ethical standards.
- *Legal and ethical guidance*: Researchers should seek legal and ethical guidance when faced with dilemmas related to disclosures. Consulting legal experts and ethics committees can help them make informed decisions while ensuring transparency.

CASE STUDY: THE WAKEFIELD MMR VACCINE CONTROVERSY[10]

A classic example of the consequences of inadequate disclosures and ethical lapses in scientific research is the Andrew Wakefield MMR (measles, mumps, and rubella) vaccine controversy. In 1998, Dr Andrew Wakefield and his colleagues published a study in The Lancet, a prestigious medical journal, suggesting a link between the MMR vaccine and autism. The study lacked a clear and transparent methodology, and the sample size was small. Furthermore, the study failed to disclose significant conflicts of interest, as Wakefield was involved in litigation against vaccine manufacturers.

The study, although limited in scope and methodology, generated significant public fear and distrust in vaccines. This led to a decline in vaccine uptake and contributed to outbreaks of preventable diseases. Subsequent research and investigations revealed the serious shortcomings of the study, and it was eventually retracted by The Lancet. Wakefield's medical license was revoked due to ethical breaches, and the study's repercussions are still felt today in the form of vaccine hesitancy.

The Wakefield case underscores the severe consequences that can result from inadequate disclosures, conflicts of interest, and ethical lapses in scientific research. It also demonstrates the importance of a thorough peer review process, which, if done rigorously, might have identified the study's flaws before publication.

UNDERSTANDING SCIENTIFIC MISCONDUCT

Scientific misconduct encompasses a range of unethical behaviors within the realm of research and publication. These behaviors violate established codes of ethics, standards, and principles that underpin the scientific process. The most common forms of scientific misconduct include:[11,12]

- *Falsification of data*: This involves manipulating, altering, or fabricating research data to support a desired outcome or conclusion. Falsification undermines the credibility of the research and can lead to erroneous conclusions.
- *Plagiarism*: It occurs when an individual uses someone else's ideas, words, or work without proper attribution. It is a breach of academic and scientific integrity that can seriously harm one's reputation.
- *Fabrication*: It goes beyond manipulating data; it involves making up data entirely. This blatant dishonesty can have severe consequences, as it misleads other researchers and the public.
- *Selective reporting*: Researchers may choose to selectively report only positive or statistically significant results while omitting less favorable findings. This can lead to a skewed understanding of the research.

- *Authorship misconduct*: Improper attribution of authorship or omitting deserving contributors from the author list is also a form of scientific misconduct. It can lead to disputes and discredit the research.
- *Conflict of interest*: Failing to disclose financial, personal, or other conflicts of interest can influence the objectivity and credibility of research findings.

WHY SCIENTIFIC MISCONDUCT OCCURS

Understanding why scientific misconduct occurs is crucial in addressing the issue. Several factors contribute to its occurrence:[13,14]

- *Pressure to publish*: The "publish or perish" culture prevalent in academia can drive researchers to prioritize quantity over quality. This pressure may lead some to cut corners, engage in unethical behavior, or rush through research to meet publication quotas.
- *Funding and career prospects*: Securing research funding and career advancement are highly competitive endeavors. Researchers facing funding challenges or career uncertainty may be more inclined to engage in misconduct to enhance their prospects.
- *Lack of oversight*: In some cases, inadequate oversight and lax institutional policies contribute to scientific misconduct. When misconduct goes unchecked, it can become more widespread.
- *Ethical erosion*: Some individuals may initially engage in minor ethical breaches that escalate into more severe misconduct over time. This "slippery slope" can gradually erode one's ethical standards.

IMPACT OF SCIENTIFIC MISCONDUCT[14-17]

The consequences of scientific misconduct are far-reaching and affect multiple stakeholders, including researchers, institutions, the scientific community, and society as a whole:

- *Loss of trust*: Scientific misconduct erodes public trust in research and science. When fraudulent research is uncovered, it tarnishes the reputation of the entire scientific community.
- *Wasted resources*: Misconduct consumes valuable time, money, and resources, diverting them away from legitimate and impactful research endeavors.
- *Harm to individuals*: Researchers found guilty of misconduct may face professional and personal repercussions, including damage to their careers and reputations.
- *Impact on policy and public health*: Misleading research can have direct implications for public policy and public health. False or manipulated data may lead to misguided decisions and detrimental consequences.

RETRACTION AS A MECHANISM FOR CORRECTING THE RECORD[18,19]

To address scientific misconduct and its consequences, one important mechanism is the retraction of scientific papers. Retraction is the formal process by which a journal or publisher withdraws a published research article. It is typically done when significant flaw or misconduct is identified in the research. Retractions serve several crucial purposes:

- *Correction of the scientific record*: Retractions correct the scientific record, acknowledging the errors or misconduct within a published paper. This ensures that future researchers are not misled by false or misleading information.
- *Accountability and transparency*: Retractions hold authors accountable for their misconduct or mistakes. They send a message that ethical breaches will not be tolerated and promote transparency in science.
- *Preventing further harm*: Retractions help prevent the dissemination of erroneous information that could have adverse consequences for policy, public health, or further research.

Retraction Process

The Committee on Publication Ethics (COPE) defines retraction of scientific papers as "a mechanism for correcting the literature and alerting readers to articles that contain such seriously flawed or erroneous content or data that their findings and conclusions cannot be relied upon."[20] The retraction process is not a one-size-fits-all procedure; it can vary between journals and publishers. However, it generally follows a set of common steps:

1. *Identification of issues*: Concerns regarding a published paper may be raised by the authors, other researchers, or readers. These concerns may relate to data manipulation, ethical breaches, or other issues.
2. *Investigation*: The journal or publisher initiates an investigation to assess the validity of the concerns. This often involves communication with the authors, experts in the field, and, in some cases, institutions where the research was conducted.
3. *Decision to retract*: If the investigation confirms the presence of significant issues, the journal's editorial board makes the decision to retract the paper. The reasons for retraction are clearly stated in the retraction notice.
4. *Publication of retraction notice*: The journal publishes a retraction notice alongside the retracted paper, explaining the reasons for retraction and providing transparency about the decision.
5. *Notification of institutions and funding agencies*: In cases of misconduct, the involved institutions and funding agencies may be notified of the retraction to take appropriate actions.

Challenges of Retraction[21]

Retraction is a necessary process, but it is not without challenges. Some of the key challenges associated with retractions include:

- *Delayed retractions*: Retractions can be delayed for various reasons, including resistance from authors or institutions, legal considerations, or the complexities of the investigation process. This delay can allow erroneous information to persist.
- *Stigma*: Authors of retracted papers may experience significant professional and personal stigma, even if the retraction is due to honest mistakes rather than misconduct.
- *Perceived bias*: Retractions can be misinterpreted as a sign of the scientific process's unreliability. However, they are an essential part of the process designed to correct the record.
- *Incomplete retractions*: In some cases, retractions may not fully correct the record, as they may omit crucial details about the issues in the research, leaving room for ambiguity.

PREVENTING SCIENTIFIC MISCONDUCT

Preventing scientific misconduct is a collective responsibility that involves various stakeholders. Some strategies to prevent misconduct include:[21,22]

- *Education and training*: Institutions and universities should prioritize education on research ethics and responsible conduct of research for both students and faculty.
- *Promoting ethical research culture*: Cultivating an ethical research culture, where integrity is valued above all, can deter misconduct.
- *Whistleblower protections*: Offering protection to individuals who report misconduct can encourage early detection and reporting.
- *Transparent reporting*: Journals should promote transparency by requiring detailed methods and data sharing, making it easier to spot irregularities.
- *Fostering a supportive environment*: Creating an environment where researchers are not under excessive pressure to publish can reduce the likelihood of misconduct.

CONCLUSION

For the scientific community to maintain its role as a trusted source of knowledge and innovation, it must prioritize the highest standards of honesty, integrity, and transparency. This includes rigorous methodological disclosures and a commitment to ethical conduct. Through these practices, we can continue to advance knowledge and address some of the world's most pressing issues with the confidence that scientific research is conducted with the utmost professionalism and accountability.

Scientific misconduct and the subsequent retraction of research papers are complex issues with significant consequences for the scientific community and society at large. While it is essential to address and correct unethical behavior, the focus should also be on preventing misconduct through education, fostering a culture of integrity, and creating an environment that supports responsible research.

As we move forward in the pursuit of scientific knowledge, it is crucial to remain vigilant in upholding the ethical principles that underpin the scientific process. By doing so, we can maintain the trust of the public, advance knowledge, and ensure that the fruits of scientific research benefit society as a whole.

REFERENCES

1. Harvard Medical School. (2024). Disclosures in Publications. Harvard Medical School. [online] Available from https://ari.hms.harvard.edu/research-influence/disclosures/disclosures-publications [Last accessed January, 2024].
2. Jenn NC. Common ethical issues in research and publication. Malays Fam Physician. 2006;1(2-3):74-6.
3. Tedersoo L, Küngas R, Oras E, Köster K, Eenmaa H, Leijen Ä, et al. Data sharing practices and data availability upon request differ across scientific disciplines. Sci Data. 2021;8(1):192.
4. Matas J. Publication and dissemination of research results. In Marusic A (Ed). A Guide to Responsible Research. Collaborative Bioethics, volume 1. Cham: Springer International Publishing; 2023. pp. 93-105.
5. Grady C, Horstmann E, Sussman JS, Hull SC. The limits of disclosure: what research subjects want to know about investigator financial interests. J Law Med Ethics. 2006;34(3):592-9.
6. Hellyer P. Conflicts of interest in scientific publications. Br Dent J. 2020;228(1):24.
7. Singhal S, Kalra BS. Publication ethics: Role and responsibility of authors. Indian J Gastroenterol. 2021;40:65-71.
8. Gasparyan AY, Ayvazyan L, Akazhanov NA, Kitas GD. Conflicts of interest in biomedical publications: considerations for authors, peer reviewers, and editors. Croat Med J. 2013;54(6):600.
9. Elsevier Journal Article Publishing Support Centre. (2023). What are Conflict of Interest Statements, Funding Source Declarations, Author Agreements/Declarations and Permission Notes? [online] Available from https://service.elsevier.com/app/answers/detail/a_id/286/supporthub/publishing/ [Last accessed January, 2024].
10. Godlee F, Smith J, Marcovitch H. Wakefield's article linking MMR vaccine and autism was fraudulent. BMJ. 2011;342:c7452.
11. Bauchner H, Fontanarosa PB, Flanagin A, Thornton J. Scientific misconduct and medical journals. JAMA. 2018;320(19):1985-7.
12. Gross C. Scientific misconduct. Annu Rev Psychol. 2016;67:693-711.
13. George E. (2023). Research misconduct: Reasons and types of research misconduct. [online] Available from https://researcher.life/blog/article/research-misconduct-reasons-and-types/ [Last accessed January, 2024].
14. National Academies of Sciences, Engineering, and Medicine; Policy and Global Affairs; Committee on Science, Engineering, Medicine, and Public Policy; Committee on Responsible Science. Understanding the Causes. Fostering Integrity in Research. Washington (DC): National Academies Press (US); 2017.

15. Mousavi T, Abdollahi M. A review of the current concerns about misconduct in medical sciences publications and the consequences. Daru. 2020;28:359-69.
16. Fanelli D. How many scientists fabricate and falsify research? A systematic review and meta-analysis of survey data. PLoS One. 2009;4(5):e5738.
17. Tarazi C. The Cost of Scientific Misconduct. Pediatr Res. 2015;78(5):482.
18. Elsevier Author Services. (2024). Paper Retraction: Meaning and Main Reasons. [online] Available from https://scientific-publishing.webshop.elsevier.com/research-process/paper-retraction-meaning-and-main-reasons/ [Last accessed January, 2024].
19. Candal-Pedreira C, Pérez-Ríos M, Ruano-Ravina A. Retraction of scientific papers: Types of retraction, consequences, and impacts. In: Faintuch J, Faintuch S (Eds). Integrity of Scientific Research. Cham: Springer; 2022.
20. COPE Council. (2019). COPE retraction guidelines. Committee on Publication Ethics. [online] Available from https://publicationethics.org/retraction-guidelines [Last accessed January, 2024].
21. Pollock NW. Retraction of scientific writing. Wilderness Environ Med. 2020;31(3):257-8.
22. Combating scientific misconduct. Nat Cell Biol. 2011;13:1.

CHAPTER 21

Artificial Intelligence-assisted Technology in Publication

Bidita Khandelwal, Aryan Prasad

INTRODUCTION

Artificial intelligence (AI)-powered text generation will change scientific publication to a great extent because the AI technologies have advanced to the level where machine-generated text can seamlessly be integrated into human generated text. But it will always be AI-assisted tools because human supervision will be mandatory despite the potential of AI. So "assisted driving" approach would be the best approach for a researcher where time-consuming tasks can be taken care of by AI. Critical thinking and problem-solving skills are requisite for research and quality scientific publication. Usage of AI and AI-assisted tools in an innovative manner can enhance an author's skill. But if these tools are used to falsify or fabricate, then the quality of publication will deteriorate and the ethics in publication will crumple. AI is significantly involved in the backstage of publication right from the beginning of writing a manuscript till the final publication and so the question arises whether AI-assisted tools lead to decline in editor's, reviewer's, and even the author's role. Gradual adoption of technology based on AI gives ample scope to leverage this benefit for the advancement of quality research publications.

HISTORY

John McCarthy first coined the term artificial intelligence in 1956 which subsequently was described as any thoughtful application of advanced computer sciences in executing processes and tasks related to intelligent human beings. Being one of the fastest growing industries, it is difficult to pinpoint the single "first" AI tool in the world of publishing. However, the most hyped and popular AI-integrated publishing tool is Grammarly, which was founded in 2009, enabling the users to improve their writing through AI and natural language processing (NLP). It enables the user to write better by identifying grammar and spelling errors, suggesting style improvements, and providing vocabulary enhancements.

DEFINITION

Institute of Electrical and Electronics Engineers defines AI as "the combination of computational processes, machines, and systems that can perform tasks that typically require human intelligence, such as visual perception, speech recognition, decision-making, and language translation. AI systems are designed to analyze data, learn from patterns, and make informed decisions, often using techniques like machine learning (ML) and deep learning. The goal of AI is to create machines that can simulate human intelligence and perform tasks in ways that mimic human reasoning and problem-solving".

In simpler terms, AI is like teaching a computer how to think and make decisions just like humans do. It is a way of making machines smart enough to understand our questions, learn from experiences, and help us do tasks that would normally need human thinking. AI can analyze information, recognize patterns, and even predict what might happen next based on what it has learned. It is like having a computer friend that can learn and help us solve problems in a clever way.

APPLICATION OF AI-ASSISTED TECHNOLOGY IN PUBLICATION

Artificial intelligence and AI-assisted tools are used in every step of publication, from the first step of problem-formulating to its publishing.

Literature Review

Literature review is a process consisting of various steps like problem-formulating, literature search, screening for inclusion, assessment of quality and data extraction, analysis, and interpretation. AI-based tools can be used in various steps of literature review. Literature review has mechanical repetitive tasks where AI tools can reduce the effort and time of the authors thus giving them more time for the other creative aspect of literature review requiring human expertise, interpretation, and analysis based on intuition.

In the first step of *problem formulation,* which requires identification and verification of research gaps, AI tools have moderate potential and human judgement remains paramount. Its role in interdisciplinary research is high but that requires programming skills. In the next step of *literature search* by different methods like database search, table-of-content scans, complementary search and citation search, AI-powered tools like Research rabbit, Rayyan, Consensus AI, Semantic Scholar, Iris AI, and PubMed (which uses AI to improve its search results) are very helpful in today's world when there is enormous literature available and rapid growth of research output as it spares domain expert authors from mechanical tasks, permitting more time and energy for cognitively demanding tasks. After literature search, *screening* involves separation of relevant papers from the rest based initially on the title and abstracts and then based on full text. AI-assisted tools are very effective in the initial screen but the full text-based screen requires human expertise. In manual screening, disagreements are encountered between the authors and AI-based tools help to improve and augment screening in such inconsistent results. The step of *data extraction* requires NLP and ML algorithms. AI-assisted tools have good potential in facilitating transfer and organization of data into corresponding repositories. WebPlot Digitizer or Graph-2-Data are specialized tools which extract data from tables or statistical plots. The final step is the *data analysis and interpretation* where review maybe elegant narratives or maybe more objective where aggregated evidence or descriptive overviews interfering with the accuracy are removed. AI-based tools are useful in the latter type of review. RevMan or the R-package-dMetar are the applications and libraries used for *theory testing* for meta-analyses.[1]

Create or Alter Images

Various AI-assisted technology are used to create or alter images in the research design or research method e.g., DALL-E, NightCafe, etc. Author should give a clear description of the content that was created or altered and explain how the tool helped in it. Improving the clarity or an image by adjustment of color balance, contrast or brightness is acceptable, but manipulating an image to obscure or edit (delete, move, or add) the content within an image might be considered as a scientific misconduct.

Proofreading and Language Editing Services

Artificial intelligence-enabled tools provide proofreading and language editing services. Role of AI-driven tools in creating quality content which can break language barriers and be free of grammatical errors is well-established. Paperpal and Writefull are two tools that offer AI-based language editing solutions for specifically designed researchers. Grammarly is for all-around editing while Wordtune for rewriting, shortening, and expanding the content. Hypotenuse AI and QuillBot.ai are AI-powered paraphrasing tools that are both accurate and efficient. They accurately capture the meaning of the original text, and can quickly rewrite it into a new sentence or paragraph.

Referencing and Citation

An important aspect of publishing is citation management and with tools like EndNote, Mendeley, and Zotero, the organization management and formatting of the references has been enabled. Scite is a free open-source AI-powered app that provides smart citations.

Plagiarism Detection

Originality of research and integrity in its content is mandatory for a quality publication. Plagiarized content not only leads to mistrust within the scientific world but is also a threat to an author's reputation. Detecting plagiarism was laborious and time-consuming before the advent of AI-based plagiarism detection software, but they fail to assure that the text is completely devoid of AI as it gives remarks as "Your text is likely to be written entirely by a human".

Several tools in the market utilize AI to detect plagiarism and ensure originality in written content including Turnitin which is a widely used plagiarism checker in educational institutions. Turnitin uses AI to compare submitted documents against a vast database of academic papers, publications, and internet sources to identify similarities and potential instances of plagiarism. Grammarly's plagiarism checker employs AI to analyze text and compare it to a large database of web pages and academic papers. Other AI-assisted tools used are Copyscape, Plagscan, Unicheck, and Detect GPT.

Open-access Publishing

Artificial intelligence has potential to improve the efficiency of the publishing industry, as starting from assisting in research to streamlining the content creation and its distribution, it has lot of avenues. Traditionally it was print and electronic media for open-access publishing and self-archiving of repositories. Open access was dependent mainly on the author's effort and willingness to share their research openly. With advent of AI-assisted tools, open-access publishing has become very effective and economical, both in terms of time and money.

Peer Review

Potential role of AI in different dimensions of the peer review process has been well-studied. AI-assisted peer review uses automated screening tools for various stages of pre-peer review, peer review and post-publication peer review. The impact of AI in this domain is restricted as there is need for domain expertise and intellectual efforts. AI has great potential in checking for formatting, plagiarism, and language, thus can play an important role in pre-peer review stage. However, when it comes to assessing the novelty, originality, relevance, and authenticity of the manuscript in the peer review stage, AI cannot contribute significantly.[2]

Reproducibility

An original work, when published, provides information which can be replicated and explored further by other researchers. This reproducibility is an important aspect of any scientific method. AI-assisted technology in publication has its own challenges when it comes to reproducibility. If an author uses source code implementing AI methods and experiments in publication, then the following points should be kept in mind so that AI-assisted publication is easily adopted by others as it would be reproducible.[3]

- It should be accessible.
- The contents should be searchable and understandable, thus should include basic metadata.
- License should be included so that the terms and conditions of using it and the extension of the software is available.
- Digital object identifier (DOI) or persistent uniform resource locators (URL) should be available for the version used.
- The reference and citation should be properly placed in the publication.
- Clear description of what context it has been used for and its foundational concepts

LIMITATIONS

Human input and review using reliable sources is required to authenticate the AI outputs. AI cannot replace a domain expert author. AI tool based on large language models relies on the information already available on internet. They are limited to the dominant language searched and trained on. The training of these tools is on easily available published data and so retraining with revised data, as it emerges, is necessary.

A temporary *limitation* is the use of AI in complex issues. The ease with which AI is used in complex strategic games shows its potential to surpass humans in problems considered intractable with computational approach.

Vulnerability of AI models to biases is another issue of concern. Human researchers are also biased but there are several mechanisms to track the bias, minimize it, and tackle individual bias ML techniques, due to its training as available data set (which is always from the past) are inherently conservative. As a result, using this tool for decision-making is very vulnerable to being biased. The population which is underrepresented in previous research and reviewers from low-income countries who are under selected, both can contribute to bias. Robot reviewer is an explainable AI used for risk of bias assessment and helps researchers to trace ratings of domain wise bias to the source full text document.

PERILS OF AI IN ACADEMIC PUBLISHING

Open AI can mix fact with fiction and thus can produce harmful and biased answers which can result in the spread of misinformation in the scientific arena. It lacks the ability to evaluate the reliability of processed information and the output generated regarding complex scientific concepts often containing errors. Biases due to AI-assisted tool are often amplified, spreads globally, and evades detection as it cannot be traced to an individual. There is increased risk of dependence on AI tools. When these tools are misused, there is no one accountable or responsible against whom legal actions can be taken. Certain publication houses have framed their policy governing AI-assisted research, however laws and regulations governing these tools are lacking.

CAN AI AND AI-ASSISTED TOOLS BE CREDITED AS A CO-AUTHOR FOR PUBLICATION?

The answer is "NO".

To be credited as a co-author, one is accountable and responsible for the accuracy, originality and integrity of the work and should have the ability to approve the final version of the manuscript. The term authorship implies responsibilities and tasks that are performed by and can be attributed to humans. At present, generative AI and AI-assisted tools do not qualify as co-author.

DO YOU NEED TO DISCLOSE THAT YOU HAVE USED AI-ASSISTED TECHNOLOGY?

The answer is both Yes and No.

Yes, if one uses large language models, e.g., BERT, GPT-3.5 during the scientific writing process, then it should be disclosed. However, the use of AI and AI-assisted tools in formal research design in research methods should be mentioned in the methodology section. If AI-assisted tool is used to create or alter images, the name of the tool, version, and extension number and the manufacture details should be mentioned.

No disclosure is required for the use of AI-assisted tools as spelling or grammar checkers or as reference manager (e.g., Zotero, EndNote, Mendeley, etc.), performing a statistical analysis by data input into an AI, taking AI-generated codes to perform statistical analysis or writing a conclusion for an original study carried out by researcher.

IN WHICH SECTION OF THE ARTICLE SHOULD ONE DISCLOSE AND THE FORMAT OF DOING SO?

Each journal has author guidelines that should be followed. As per Elsevier, the authors should insert a statement at the end of their manuscript, immediately above the references, entitled "Declaration of Generative AI and AI-assisted Technologies in the Writing Process". The format of the statement should be as *"During the preparation of this work the author(s) used (name tool/service) in order to (reason). After using this tool/service, the author(s) reviewed and edited the content as needed and take(s) full responsibility for the content of the publication".*

Who is the owner of the AI-generated scientific content which is the product of training over human-generated original content?

The answer to it is debatable. But as the authorship belongs to humans, so they are the owner of the content.

ACCEPTANCE OF AI-ASSISTED TECHNOLOGY

Undoubtedly, such AI-assisted approaches in publication will be met with enthusiasm by some and with reservations by some. The differing level of acceptance is well-captured in the perspectives of two scientists. According to Ray Kurzweil, thanks to AI, by 2045 "we will have multiplied the human intelligence of our civilization a billion-fold".[4] But according to Stephen Hawking, "The development of full AI could spell the end of the human race".[5] An analogy can be drawn by seeing the present-day role of calculators in mathematics. When calculators first came in the market, there was apprehension that it would threaten the training in mathematics. But the adaptation of calculators made it an integral part in training and application of mathematics.

CONCLUSION

Artificial intelligence and AI-assisted technologies are to be used in improving the language and readability but not to replace the skills of an author in providing medical and scientific insights or giving clinical recommendations. There are several concerns and perils with AI-assisted tools but these can be mitigated by small adjustments and in some by systemic changes. Adjustment and adaptation will help to reap maximum benefit and restrict use of tools which are still unreliable. Generative AI tools have revolutionized publication and its various aspects but there are several challenges related to practical aspects, moral and ethical issues and policy related to its uses. There is vast opportunity to leverage AI in support of various research tasks. AI has great potential in repetitive tasks but in tasks requiring interpretation and analysis, the potential varies from moderate to nil. With great infrastructure and conducive environment, one needs to learn the right skills, have a vision, devote time, have commitment, patience, and dedication, only then one can harness the best potential of AI-assisted technology.

TAKE-HOME MESSAGES

- AI-assisted technology has great potential in scientific publication.
- Gradual adoption of AI-based tools integrated with the human domain expertise is the need of the hour.
- Author should be aware of the limitation and the bias of the tool in order to leverage its best potential.
- AI-assisted technology cannot be credited as a co-author.

REFERENCES

1. Wagner G, Lukyanenko R, Paré G. Artificial intelligence and the conduct of literature reviews. J Inf Technol. 2021;37(2):209-26.
2. Spezi V, Wakeling S, Pinfield S, Fry J, Creaser C, Willett P. Let the community decide? The vision and reality of soundness only peer review in open-access mega-journals. J Doc. 2018;74:137-61.
3. Gundersen OF, Gil Y, Aha DW. On Reproducible AI: Towards Reproducible Research, Open Science, and Digital Scholarship in AI Publications. AI Magazine. 2018;39:56-68.
4. Reedy C. (2017). Kurzweil claims that the singularity will happen by 2045: Get ready for humanity 2.0. [online] Available from https://futurism.com/kurzweil-claims-that-the-singularity-will-happen-by-2045 [Last accessed January, 2024].
5. AIReligion. Stephen Hawking warns artificial intelligence may supersede humans, disrupt economy. [online] Available from [Last accessed January, 2024].

Self-Assessment

1. **What is IMRAD format?**
2. **Which abbreviation is used for objective framing?**
3. **What is the common style of referencing used in medical journals?**
4. **Which referencing style follows alphabetical order?**
5. **What is the most important step in the publication of an image-based article?**
   a. To have an idea whether the image is publishable or not.
   b. To take assistance from ChatGPT.
   c. To use a good-quality image.
   d. To prepare the manuscript in a sequential manner.
6. **Common factors that lead to rejection are all *except*:**
   a. Insufficient quality of image
   b. Lack of context and novelty
   c. Ethical concerns
   d. None of the above
7. **The steps to be followed for preparation for the publication of a clinical image-based article include:**
   a. Selecting the right journal
   b. Your article aligns with the journal's scope and formatting guidelines
   c. Images for the article should be of optimum quality
   d. All of the above
8. **Qualities of a good-quality clinical image include all *except*:**
   a. High-resolution images with clear focus and proper lighting.
   b. Patient identity remains protected, with no identifying features or information visible in the image.
   c. Inappropriate patient positioning.
   d. An image with a neutral, uncluttered background that eliminates distractions and keeps the focus on the clinical subject.
9. **The preparation and publication of a "starry sky appearance of tuberculoma" include the following *except*:**
   a. Preparation of the manuscript in the following order: History, examination, investigations, treatment, differential, and final diagnosis followed by discussion.
   b. The discussion should be referenced properly.
   c. The MRI plate is to be put in the view box and the image should be clicked.
   d. Written informed consent is to be taken.

10. The letter must be an elaborate discussion of a published article/scientific discourse. (True/False)

11. Letter to the editor is a direct communication between the reader and author. (True/False)

12. In no way, the letter to the editor helps a novel researcher. (True/False)

13. The language in the letter must be courteous and polite. (True/False)

14. As it is in the form of a letter, it should be devoid of any title. (True/False)

15. Reporting guidelines for systematic reviews and meta-analysis are called:

a. ARRIVE
b. CONSORT
c. PRISMA
d. STROBE

16. Authorship of biomedical publications requires mandatory contribution toward all *except*:

a. Arrangement of funding for the project
b. Drafting or revising the work for intellectual content
c. Final approval of the version to be published
d. Taking public responsibility for the work

17. The CONSORT guidelines checklist encourages all *except*:

a. Disclosure of the source of funding
b. Statement of statistical analysis plan
c. Disclosure of ethical safeguards used in the study
d. Structured abstract covering trial design, methods, results, and conclusions

18. In general, pharmaceutical products used in clinical research should be named by their:

a. Chemical name
b. International nonproprietary name
c. International trade name
d. Actual brand name

19. Which of the following is NOT a feature of the Vancouver style of referencing?

a. It is a numerical referencing style.
b. Author names have to be cited in the main text.
c. References are arranged in order of their occurrence in the text.
d. Journal names are abbreviated in a standard manner.

20. A case report usually a word limit of:

a. 1,000–1,500
b. 1,500–2,000
c. 2,000–2,500
d. 2,500–3,000

21. A case series comprises:

a. 1–4 Cases
b. 4–10 Cases
c. 10–15 Cases
d. None of the above

22. Word limit excludes:

a. Abstract
b. References
c. Both abstract and references
d. None of the above

23. **Reporting guidelines for case reports are the:**
    a. CONSORT guidelines
    b. PRISMA guidelines
    c. CARE guidelines
    d. STROBE guidelines

24. **Creative commons attribution non-commercial refers to:**
    a. License to share information
    b. License to adapt
    c. License to build upon
    d. All of the above
    e. None of the above

25. **Abstract all are true *except*:**
    a. Concise and short
    b. Word limit - 250–350
    c. Abbreviations may be used
    d. May be unstructured

26. **Consent of patient–all are true *except*:**
    a. It is optional
    b. Uploading of consent is optional
    c. Relative can give consent
    d. Patient can read the manuscript

27. **Original articles - all are true *except*:**
    a. Primary literature
    b. Secondary literature
    c. Require IRB approval
    d. Includes systematic review articles

28. **Sample size calculation is by:**
    a. Cochran's formula
    b. Smidt's formula
    c. Manden's formula
    d. Toren's formula

29. **What is the value of Z-score in a 95% confidence limit for sample size calculation?**
    a. 1.26
    b. 1.96
    c. 1.76
    d. None of the above

30. **References are not given in:**
    a. Introduction
    b. Methodology
    c. Results
    d. Discussion

31. **All are true about text, *except*:**
    a. Number less than ten in words
    b. Number more the ten in digits
    c. Number less than one start with a zero
    d. Give a space between number and percentage sign

32. **IMRAD includes all *except*:**
    a. Introduction
    b. Methodology
    c. Results
    d. Analysis
    e. Discussion

33. **Fabrication and falsification - all are true *except*:**
    a. Are synonymous
    b. Not synonymous
    c. Type of plagiarism
    d. Unethical

34. Salami slicing all are true *except*:
a. Unethical
b. Multiple papers with same population
c. Same data set
d. Different hypothesis

35. Number of references in original articles:
a. 10–20
b. 20–50
c. 50–100

36. All are true about data sharing *except*:
a. Participant data after deidentification may be shared
b. Statistical analysis report
c. Informed consent form
d. Available 3 months before publication

37. Direct quoting, paraphrasing or a summary are all allowed in 'in-text citation'.
a. Agree
b. Disagree

38. In text reference should be put at the end of a sentence (may be also in the middle of a sentence)
a. Agree
b. Disagree

39. A Vancouver reference list is arranged alphabetically:
a. Agree
b. Disagree

40. Year of publication follows the name of authors in Harvard style of citation:
a. Agree
b. Disagree

41. A digital object identifier (DOI) is the address of a given unique resource on the web/webpage:
a. Agree
b. Disagree

42. Citation of a book chapter is same as that of an article in a journal:
a. Agree
b. Disagree

43. Duplication of reference may occur in citation management software:
a. Agree
b. Disagree

44. The *h*-index denotes the status of the journal:
a. Agree
b. Disagree

45. Impact factor calculation considers 4 years of citations:
a. Agree
b. Disagree

46. It is good to include as many references as possible to signify a well researched article:
a. Agree
b. Disagree

State whether the following statements are True (T) or False (F)

47. Higher the impact factor, higher chance of acceptance of your article. T/F

48. Open access journals provide broader readership. T/F

49. Avoid journals with rigorous peer review – high chance of rejection. T/F

50. **Predatory journals have high publication fees. T/F**
51. **It is not necessary to answer to each and every author query. T/F**
52. **A conflict of interest statement means a disagreement among authors. T/F**
53. **A consent letter is not mandatory for case reports. T/F**
54. **The correct term is Ethical Committee Clearance. T/F**
55. **What is the major role of AI in literature search?**
56. **To serve what purpose should AI be actually used in publication?**
57. **Who coined the term "Artificial Intelligence" and when?**
58. **Which segment of the AI tool is most commonly used and observed in assistance to publication?**
59. **Who owns AI-generated scientific content?**

Answers

1. IMRAD structure stands for introduction, methodology, results and discussion.
2. Objective framing 'SMART' specific, measurable, attainable, relevant, time-bound.

3. Vancouver style	4. Harvard	5. a	6. d
7. d	8. c	9. c	10. False
11. False	12. False	13. True	14. False
15. c	16. a	17. b	18. b
19. b	20. a	21. b	22. c
23. c	24. d	25. c	26. a
27. b	28. a	29. b	30. c
31. d	32. d	33. b	34. d
35. b	36. d	37. Agree	38. Disagree
39. Disagree	40. Agree		

41. Disagree – locates a particular article not webpage 42. Disagree
43. Agree 44. Disagree 45. Disagree
46. Disagree – specified no is given in instructions to authors
47. False – high rejection rate 48. True
49. False – it increases the credibility of the your desirable
50. False – nominal fees usually 51. False – answer all queries
52. False – means the author may have some financial/personal gains from the study 53. False – mandatory
54. False – Ethics Committee approval 55. Enhancement
56. Improvement 57. John McCarthy in 1956
58. Plagiarism checker 59. Humans

INDEX

Page numbers followed by *b* refer to box.